Evaluation of the Small Bowel

Editor

LAUREN B. GERSON

GASTROINTESTINAL ENDOSCOPY CLINICS OF NORTH AMERICA

www.giendo.theclinics.com

Consulting Editor
CHARLES J. LIGHTDALE

January 2017 • Volume 27 • Number 1

ELSEVIER

1600 John F. Kennedy Boulevard • Suite 1800 • Philadelphia, Pennsylvania, 19103-2899

http://www.theclinics.com

GASTROINTESTINAL ENDOSCOPY CLINICS OF NORTH AMERICA Volume 27, Number 1
January 2017 ISSN 1052-5157, ISBN-13: 978-0-323-48260-8

Editor: Kerry Holland
Developmental Editor: Donald Mumford

Gastrointestinal Endoscopy Clinics of North America (ISSN 1052-5157) is published quarterly by Elsevier Inc., 360 Park Avenue South, New York, NY 10010-1710. Months of issue are January, April, July, and October. Business and Editorial Offices: 1600 John F. Kennedy Blvd., Suite 1800, Philadelphia, PA, 19103-2899. Periodicals postage paid at New York, NY and additional mailing offices. Subscription prices are $342.00 per year for US individuals, $560.00 per year for US institutions, $100.00 per year for US students and residents, $377.00 per year for Canadian individuals, $662.00 per year for Canadian institutions, $474.00 per year for international individuals, $662.00 per year for international institutions, and $245.00 per year for Canadian and foreign students/residents. To receive student/resident rate, orders must be accompanied by name of affiliated institution, date of term, and the *signature* of program/residency coordinator on institution letterhead. Orders will be billed at individual rate until proof of status is received. Foreign air speed delivery is included in all *Clinics* subscription prices. All prices are subject to change without notice. **POSTMASTER:** Send address change to *Gastrointestinal Endoscopy Clinics of North America*, Elsevier Health Sciences Division, Subscription Customer Service, 3251 Riverport Lane, Maryland Heights, MO 63043. **Customer Service: 1-800-654-2452 (US). From outside the United States, call 1-314-447-8871. Fax: 1-314-447-8029. E-mail: JournalsCustomerService-usa@elsevier.com (for print support) or JournalsOnlineSupport-usa@elsevier.com (for online support).**

Reprints. For copies of 100 or more, of articles in this publication, please contact the Commercial Reprints Department, Elsevier Inc., 360 Park Avenue South, New York, NY 10010-1710. Tel. 212-633-3874; Fax: 212-633-3820; E-mail: reprints@elsevier.com.

Gastrointestinal Endoscopy Clinics of North America is covered in *Excerpta Medica, MEDLINE/PubMed (Index Medicus), and MEDLINE/MEDLARS.*

Contributors

CONSULTING EDITOR

CHARLES J. LIGHTDALE, MD
Professor of Medicine, Division of Digestive and Liver Diseases, Columbia University
Medical Center, New York, New York

EDITOR

LAUREN B. GERSON, MD, MSc
Director of Clinical Research, Gastroenterology Fellowship Program, California Pacific
Medical Center, Associate Clinical Professor of Medicine, University of California
San Francisco, San Francisco, California

AUTHORS

JAMES C. ANDREWS, MD
Professor, Department of Radiology, Mayo Clinic, Rochester, Minnesota

JAMIE S. BARKIN, MD, MACG, MACP, AGAF, FASGE
Professor of Medicine, Division of Gastroenterology, Department of Medicine, Leonard M.
Miller School of Medicine, University of Miami, Miami, Florida

JODIE A. BARKIN, MD
Gastroenterology Fellow, Division of Gastroenterology, Department of Medicine, Leonard
M. Miller School of Medicine, University of Miami, Miami, Florida

ANNE BERGER, MD
Department of General and Digestive Surgery, Georges Pompidou European AP-HP
University Hospital; Paris Descartes Faculty of Medicine, Paris, France

STEPHANE BONNET, MD
Department of Digestive Surgery, Percy University Military Hospital, Clamart, France

CHRISTOPHE CELLIER, MD, PhD
Department of Gastroenterology and Endoscopy, Georges Pompidou European AP-HP
University Hospital; Paris Descartes Faculty of Medicine, Paris, France

DIRK DOMAGK, MD, FASGE
Professor of Medicine; Head, Department of Medicine I, Josephs-Hospital Warendorf,
Academic Teaching Hospital, University of Muenster, Warendorf, Germany

RICHARD DOUARD, MD, PhD
Department of General and Digestive Surgery, Georges Pompidou European AP-HP
University Hospital; Paris Descartes Faculty of Medicine, Paris, France

JEFF L. FIDLER, MD
Professor, Department of Radiology, Mayo Clinic, Rochester, Minnesota

CHAD J. FLEMING, MD
Assistant Professor, Department of Radiology, Mayo Clinic, Rochester, Minnesota

JULIO GEORGIOU, PhD, DIC, MEng
Department of Electrical and Computer Engineering, University of Cyprus, Aglantzia, Cyprus

LAUREN B. GERSON, MD, MSc
Director of Clinical Research, Gastroenterology Fellowship Program, California Pacific Medical Center, Associate Clinical Professor of Medicine, University of California San Francisco, San Francisco, California

AJIT H. GOENKA, MD
Assistant Professor, Department of Radiology, Mayo Clinic, Rochester, Minnesota

CHRISTIAN S. JACKSON, MD, FACG
Chief, Section of Gastroenterology, VA Loma Linda Healthcare System, Loma Linda, California

ANASTASIOS KOULAOUZIDIS, MD, FACG, FEBG, FRCPE
Centre for Liver and Digestive Disorders, The Royal Infirmary of Edinburgh, Edinburgh, United Kingdom

BRIAN LACY, MD, PhD
Division of Gastroenterology and Hepatology, Dartmouth-Hitchcock Medical Center, Lebanon, New Hampshire

DANIEL A. LEFFLER, MD, MS
Division of Gastroenterology, The Celiac Center, Beth Israel Deaconess Medical Center, Boston, Massachusetts

JONATHAN A. LEIGHTON, MD
Division of Gastroenterology and Hepatology, Scottsdale, Arizona

PHILIPP LENZ, MD
Department of Palliative Care, Institute of Palliative Care, University Hospital of Muenster, Muenster, Germany

GEORGIA MALAMUT, MD, PhD
Department of Gastroenterology and Endoscopy, Georges Pompidou European AP-HP University Hospital; Paris Descartes Faculty of Medicine, Paris, France

ANDREA MAY, MD
Department of Gastroenterology, Sana Klinikum Offenbach GmbH, Offenbach am Main, Germany

SHABANA F. PASHA, MD
Division of Gastroenterology and Hepatology, Mayo Clinic, Scottsdale, Arizona

MARCO PENNAZIO, MD
Head; Small-Bowel Diseases Unit, Division of Gastroenterology U, San Giovanni AS University-Teaching Hospital, Torino, Italy

GABRIEL RAHMI, MD, PhD
Department of Gastroenterology and Endoscopy, Georges Pompidou European AP-HP University Hospital; Paris Descartes Faculty of Medicine, Paris, France

REDDY SUREKHA, MBChB, MRCS, MD, FRCR
Department of Radiology, Western General Hospital, Edinburgh, United Kingdom

EMANUELE RONDONOTTI, MD, PhD
Gastroenterology Unit, Valduce Hospital, Como, Italy

SARAH SHANNAHAN, MD
Division of Internal Medicine, Beth Israel Deaconess Medical Center, Boston, Massachusetts

RICHARD STRONG, MD, FACG
Section of Gastroenterology, VA Loma Linda Healthcare System, Loma Linda, California

NEIL VOLK, MD
Division of Gastroenterology and Hepatology, Dartmouth-Hitchcock Medical Center, Lebanon, New Hampshire

THIBAULT VORON, MD
Department of General and Digestive Surgery, Georges Pompidou European AP-HP University Hospital; Paris Descartes Faculty of Medicine, Paris, France

PHILIPPE WIND, MD
Department of Digestive Surgery, Avicenne AP-HP University Hospital; UFR SMBH, Paris-Nord University, Bobigny, France

DIANA E. YUNG, MBChB
Centre for Liver and Digestive Disorders, The Royal Infirmary of Edinburgh, Edinburgh, United Kingdom

Contents

Comprehension of small intestine physiology and function provides a
framework for the understanding of several important disease pathways
of the gastrointestinal system. This article reviews the development, anatomy and histology of the small bowel in addition to physiology and digestion of key nutrients.

Video capsule endoscopy (VCE) has completed the endoscopic visualization of the entire luminal gastrointestinal tract. VCE can be performed in inpatients and outpatients, requires appropriate bowel preparation before
the study, and can be administered via oral swallowing or endoscopic device placement into the small bowel based on outlined patient-dependent
factors. Current commercially available VCE systems were reviewed and
compared for individual features and attributes. This article focuses on
preparation for VCE, currently available VCE technology, how to read a
VCE study, and risks and contraindications to VCE.

Small bowel capsule endoscopy (SBCE) remains the gold standard for the
diagnosis of small bowel disorders. A rather challenging task, for those
who start to use this diagnostic modality, is the recognition of the typical
anatomic landmarks and the distinction of normal small bowel anatomy
from abnormal findings. The reader of SBCE images may also often
encounter unusual views of the normal anatomy as well as various artifacts
that need to be distinguished from pathologic findings. Experience gained
through standard endoscopy is invaluable to the interpretation of capsule
examinations; however, formalized training and credentialing in reading
competency are essential.

Gastrointestinal angiodysplasia (GIAD) are red flat arborized lesions that are found throughout the entire gastrointestinal tract. GIAD can vary in size and have a range of presentation from occult to life-threatening bleeding. The typical presentation is intermittent bleeding in the setting of iron deficiency anemia. Endoscopy is the primary means of diagnosis and endoscopic therapy is noted to be initially effective. However, rebleeding can be as high as 40% to 50% in patients with small bowel GIAD. This review describes the pathophysiology for the development of GIAD and the current roles of endoscopic, medical, and surgical therapy in its treatment.

The most common small bowel inflammatory disorders include Crohn disease, nonsteroidal antiinflammatory drug (NSAID) enteropathy, and celiac disease. Capsule endoscopy, computed tomography enterography, and magnetic resonance enterography have a complementary role in the diagnosis of Crohn disease and evaluation of patients with established Crohn disease. The higher risk of capsule retention with known Crohn disease and NSAID enteropathy can be minimized by cross-sectional imaging or the patency capsule. The main role of deep enteroscopy is tissue diagnosis, endoscopic management of small bowel lesions and strictures, and retrieval of retained capsules.

Celiac disease is an autoimmune disorder induced by gluten in genetically susceptible individuals. It can result in intraintestinal and extraintestinal manifestations of disease including diarrhea, weight loss, anemia, osteoporosis, or lymphoma. Diagnosis of celiac disease is made through initial serologic testing and then confirmed by histopathologic examination of duodenal biopsies. Generally celiac disease is a benign disorder with a good prognosis in those who adhere to a gluten-free diet. However, in refractory disease, complications may develop that warrant additional testing with more advanced radiologic and endoscopic methods. This article reviews the current strategy to diagnose celiac disease and the newer modalities to assess for associated complications.

The incidence of small bowel tumors is increasing over time. Until recently, their diagnosis was delayed and it was often reached only at the time of surgery. New diagnostic tools, such as capsule endoscopy, device-assisted enteroscopy, and dedicated small bowel cross-sectional imaging techniques, have been introduced recently in clinical practice. The combination of these tools allows medical practitioners to detect small bowel tumors at an early stage and to reach a definite diagnosis before surgery, thus enabling minimally invasive treatments.

Since the introduction of double-balloon enteroscopy 15 years ago, flexible enteroscopy has become an established method in the diagnostic and therapeutic work-up of small bowel disorders. With appropriate patient selection, diagnostic and therapeutic yields of 70% to 85% can be expected. The complication rates with diagnostic and therapeutic DBE are estimated at approximately 1% and 3% to 4%, respectively. Appropriate patient selection and device selection, as well as skill, are the key issues for successful enteroscopy. However, technical developments and improvements mean that carrying out enteroscopy is likely to become easier.

Single-balloon enteroscopy is among 3 device-assisted enteroscopy systems on the market. Compared with double-balloon enteroscopy, no significant difference in diagnostic yield was found. Additionally, no significant difference was found in oral and anal insertion depth, adverse events, or procedure times. Some studies observed lower complete enteroscopy rates, which have evidently no diagnostic impact. With a learning curve of around 30 procedures, the single-balloon endoscope is a safe endoscopic tool, which seems equally suitable for diagnostic and therapeutic interventions. Carbon dioxide should be used for single-balloon endoscopy procedures, especially in patients with a history of surgical abdominal interventions.

Radiology examinations play a major role in the diagnosis, management, and surveillance of small bowel diseases and are complementary to endoscopic techniques. Computed tomography enterography and magnetic resonance enterography are the cross-sectional imaging studies of choice for many small bowel diseases. Angiography still plays an important role for catheter-directed therapies. With the emergence of hybrid imaging techniques, radionuclide imaging has shown promise for the evaluation of small bowel bleeding and Crohn disease and may play a larger role in the future. This article reviews recent advances in technology, diagnosis, and therapeutic options for selected small bowel disorders.

Intraoperative enteroscopy (IOE) to explore obscure gastrointestinal bleeding is now rarely indicated. IOE allows complete small bowel exploration in 57% to 100% of cases, finds a bleeding source in 80% of cases, allows the recurrence-free management of gastrointestinal bleeding in 76% of cases, but carries a high morbidity and mortality. IOE only remains indicated to guide the intraoperative treatment of preoperatively identified small bowel lesions when nonoperative treatments are unavailable and/or when intraoperative localization by external examination is impossible.

Patients previously classified with "obscure gastrointestinal hemorrhage" should now be classified as "suspected small bowel bleeding" according to the 2015 American College of Gastroenterology guidelines. This article provides algorithms for how to manage patients with suspected small bowel bleeding, including utilization of second-look endoscopy and/or colonoscopy, video capsule endoscopy, computed tomographic enterography, magnetic resonance enterography, angiography, and deep enteroscopy.

GASTROINTESTINAL ENDOSCOPY CLINICS OF NORTH AMERICA

RELATED INTEREST

Gastroenterology Clinics of North America, September 2016, (Vol. 45, No. 3)
Gastrointestinal Neoplasia
Paul J. Limburg and Dan A. Dixon, *Editors*

THE CLINICS ARE AVAILABLE ONLINE!
Access your subscription at:
www.theclinics.com

GASTROINTESTINAL ENDOSCOPY CLINICS
OF NORTH AMERICA

FORTHCOMING ISSUES

April 2017
Bariatric and Metabolic Endoscopy
Richard I. Rothstein, Editor

July 2017
New Directions in Interventional Endoscopy
Nicholas J. Shaheen, Editor

October 2017
...

RECENT ISSUES

October 2016
Endoscopy in Inflammatory Bowel Disease
Maria T. Abreu, Editor

July 2016
Sedation and Monitoring in Gastrointestinal
Endoscopy
John J. Vargo, Editor

Foreword

Small Intestine: Exploring the Last Great Frontier for Gastrointestinal Endoscopy

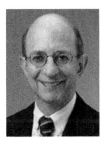

Charles J. Lightdale, MD
Consulting Editor

The small intestine—with its daunting length and sharp turns—was an impossible barrier to cross in early gastrointestinal endoscopy. The emerging technologies of video capsule endoscopy and deep enteroscopy have now provided the cameras and guns for increasing numbers of inveterate gastrointestinal endoscopists to explore the entire dimensions of this last frontier. It's still a wild space to map, but the need to do so is evident. Bleeding from the small intestine is on the rise probably related to many factors, including longer life spans, associated heart and kidney disease, nonsteroidal anti-inflammatory drugs, and anticoagulation. Inflammatory bowel disease and celiac disease are on an uptick, and while small bowel neoplasia is uncommon, diagnosis can pose a major problem. Important new radiologic tools are also now available to bolster endoscopic exploration, including computer tomographic enteroscopy and angiography and magnetic resonance enterography.

This issue of *Gastrointestinal Endoscopy Clinics of North America* on the "Evaluation of the Small Intestine" is a remarkable and comprehensive presentation of the state-of-the-art. Dr Lauren Gerson, the editor for this issue and a renowned leader in gastroenterology, has selected topics that truly cover the field and are written by an outstanding group of authors. The issue begins with a terrific review of the anatomy and physiology of the small bowel, essential information for any endoscopic explorer. Reviews follow on video capsule technique and interpretation, double-balloon enteroscopy, and single-balloon enteroscopy. The key diseases of the small bowel are covered in great detail: angiodysplasia, inflammatory disorders, celiac disease, and neoplastic diseases. The roles of radiologic techniques and intraoperative enteroscopy are thoroughly presented as well. Finally, in a superb coda, there is an updated, invaluable algorithm and outcomes discussion for small bowel bleeding.

Gastrointest Endoscopy Clin N Am 27 (2017) xiii–xiv
http://dx.doi.org/10.1016/j.giec.2016.11.001
1052-5157/17/© 2016 Published by Elsevier Inc.

Gastroenterologists, surgeons, radiologists, listen up—the small intestine frontier is open and teamwork is mandatory. It all becomes clear in this issue of the *Gastrointestinal Endoscopy Clinics of North America*.

Charles J. Lightdale, MD
Department of Medicine
Columbia University Medical Center
161 Fort Washington Avenue
New York, NY 10032, USA

E-mail address:
CJL18@columbia.edu

Preface

Evaluation of the Small Intestine

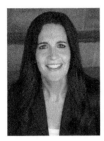

Lauren B. Gerson, MD, MSc
Editor

Evaluation of the small bowel has been traditionally challenging due to the length of the small intestine and difficulty with access other than by operative means. Introduction of video capsule endoscopy (VCE) and deep enteroscopy in the early 2000s has allowed physicians to visualize the entirely of the small bowel and perform therapeutic maneuvers. Despite these advances, patients with bleeding or other abnormalities of the small bowel remain more difficult to diagnose and treat compared to patients with disorders in the upper or lower gastrointestinal tracts. Consequently, these patients have accrued greater medical costs and longer hospital stays. While it is unclear at the present time whether evaluation with VCE and/or deep enteroscopy has reduced overall costs for patients with small bowel disorders, we have learned that use of these tools early in the presentation of suspected small bowel bleeding is associated with higher diagnostic yields. With the advent of computed tomographic enterography (CTE) and MRI enterography (MRE), pathologic findings that are extraluminal can now often be detected, increasing the diagnostic yield for patients with normal endoscopic examinations. In addition, CTE and MRE have greatly enhanced our ability to characterize inflammatory lesions of the small bowel with more accuracy. For patients with massive suspected small bowel bleeding, use of CT angiography prior to angiography has enhanced the interventional radiologist's ability to detect bleeding sources and direct subsequent angiographic intervention.

This issue of *Gastrointestinal Endoscopy Clinics of North America* presents articles on anatomy and physiology of the small bowel, technical aspects associated with reading of VCE studies, photodocumentation of normal and abnormal findings on VCE, including vascular findings, inflammatory and neoplastic disorders, and celiac disease. There is an additional article focusing on outcomes and treatment options for patients with small bowel angiodysplastic lesions. Subsequent articles describe double- and single-balloon enteroscopy, when and how to perform radiologic examinations, including CT and MR enterography, angiography, and nuclear medicine studies, and potential roles for intraoperative enteroscopy. The final article focuses on updated algorithms for patients with suspected small bowel bleeding. Given the

Gastrointest Endoscopy Clin N Am 27 (2017) xv–xvi
http://dx.doi.org/10.1016/j.giec.2016.09.001
1052-5157/17/© 2016 Published by Elsevier Inc.

giendo.theclinics.com

technological advances in small bowel imaging, the term "obscure gastrointestinal bleeding" has now been reserved for patients with suspected small bowel bleeding and normal findings on VCE, enteroscopy, enterography, and other diagnostic examinations.

Lauren B. Gerson, MD, MSc
California Pacific Medical Center
University of California, San Francisco
San Francisco, CA 94115, USA

E-mail address:
lgersonmd@yahoo.com

Anatomy and Physiology of the Small Bowel

Neil Volk, MD*, Brian Lacy, MD, PhD

KEYWORDS

- Embryology • Enteric nervous system • Small intestine • Villi • Anatomy • Digestion
- Physiology

KEY POINTS

- Embryologically, weeks 9 and 10 are critical time points with the potential for development of malrotation.
- Abnormalities in neural crest cell migration during the first trimester may lead to various neuropathies, one of the most common being Hirshsprung disease.
- The enteric nervous system plays a critical role in gut motility, secretion, and immune function.

EMBRYOLOGY
Development of Morphologic Structures

A review of the gut embryologic process provides a framework for understanding the function of the small bowel as well as the pathways that may lead to small intestinal disease. For the purpose of this review, the development of the small intestine is briefly examined with a focus on the major events outlined in **Table 1**.

Morphogenesis begins with gastrulation, the process of cell migration through the primitive streak, with eventual formation of the three fundamental germ layers of the embryo: ectoderm, mesoderm and endoderm. Although the small intestine is composed of cells that originate in all 3 layers, it is from the endoderm that the gastrointestinal (GI) tract initially develops and ultimately gives rise to the epithelium of the GI tract.[1]

The intestinal lumen first takes the form of an elementary tube during the fourth week of embryogenesis when the cranial, lateral and caudal edges of the trilaminar embryonic disk fold under the dorsal axial structures and are brought together along the now ventral surface of the embryo. The process of tube formation is mediated by several genes, including GATA4, FOXA2, and SOX9.[2] The assignment of biologic fate

The authors have no financial or nonfinancial interests to disclose.
Division of Gastroenterology and Hepatology, Dartmouth-Hitchcock Medical Center, 1 Medical Center Drive, Lebanon, NH, USA
* Corresponding author.
E-mail address: Neil.Volk@hitchcock.org

Table 1 Key events in the embryogenesis of the small intestine	
Weeks	**Major Developmental Milestones**
3	Gastrulation: Early tubular gut formation; early formation of major digestive glands
4	Gut tube closes
5	Intestinal loop beginning to form
7	Herniation of intestinal loop
8	Intestine rotates in a counterclockwise direction and recanalizes; early innervation of parasympathetic neural precursors
9	Herniated gut returns into body cavity; epithelial cells differentiate
11	Small intestine begins to develop villi; goblet cells differentiate
12	Intestinal enzymes present
20	Peyer patches seen in small intestine

to small intestine cells, a process called specification, is triggered by CDXC.[3] The acquisition of specialized features of the small intestine is dependent on interactions between the endoderm and mesoderm via the Hox signaling pathway. The resulting simple tubular structure consists of two blind ends on the cranial and caudal sides representing the foregut and hindgut, respectively. Between these two blind ends resides the future midgut. At this stage, the midgut remains largely open to the yolk sac, which has grown at a slower rate than the embryo. As development continues, the edges of the embryonic disc fuse together with the lateral margins of the midgut, forming a lumen, while the prior open connection to the yolk sac is reduced to a narrow tube called the vitelline duct.[4]

In the fifth week, the midgut has elongated to such a degree that it is forced to fold, thus forming the primary intestinal loop; by the sixth week, this loop herniates through the umbilicus (**Fig. 1**). Herniation of the bowel wall is necessary because the length of the gut increases faster than the length of the embryo and due to crowding by the proportionally larger liver and kidneys at this stage of development. The developing intestinal tract returns to the abdominal cavity between weeks 9 to 10 when the abdominal cavity is large enough to accommodate the intestinal tract.[5] During the process of herniation, the intestinal loop rotates counterclockwise 90°, resulting in an ileum that lies in the right abdomen. As the intestinal loop returns into the abdominal cavity, it rotates an additional 180° counterclockwise, resulting in the final configuration of the gut in the abdominal cavity. This process is complete by week 11.

Formation of Villi

The villi of the small intestine form from simple epithelium during week 11. Villi and crypts develop in a coordinated manner, because villi formation is accompanied by invagination into the mesoderm, which eventually forms the intestinal crypts. This process is in part mediated by Shh and Ihh.[6] Beginning during early development, and progressing through adulthood, the epithelial cells of the small intestine need to be constantly replaced due to frequent turnover. Stem cells located at the base of intestinal crypts are integral to this process. Stem cells generate progenitors for the epithelial cells lining the small intestine, a process mediated by several important signaling pathways including Wnt, Notch, and hedgehog.[7–9] As these cells mature, they migrate up the villus, where they eventually interface with the intestinal lumen.

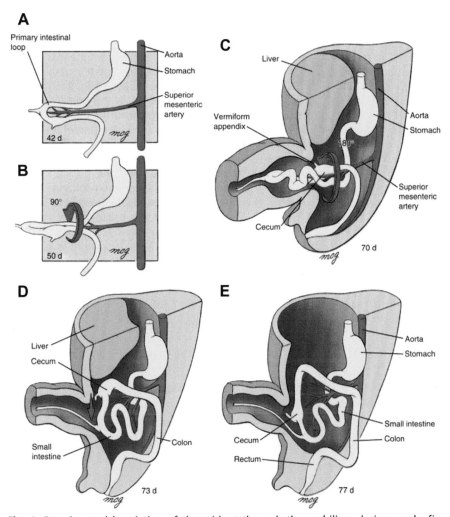

Fig. 1. Rotation and herniation of the midgut through the umbilicus during weeks five through six. (*A* and *B*) At the end of the sixth week, the primary intestinal loop herniates into the umbilicus, rotating through 90 degrees counterclockwise. (*C*) The small intestine elongates to form jejunalileal loops, the cecum and appendix grow, and at the end of the tenth week, the primary intestinal loops retracts into the abdominal cavity, rotating an additional 180 degrees counterclockwise. (*D* and *E*) During the eleventh week, the re-tracting midgut completes this rotation as the cecum is positioned just inferior to the liver. The cecum is then displaced inferiorly, pulling down the proximal hindgut to form the ascending colon. The descending colon is simultaneously fixed on the lest side of the pos-terior abdominal wall. The jejunum, ileum, transverse colon, and gigmoid colon remain sus-pended by mesentery. (*From* Schoenwolf GC, Larsen WJ. Larsen's human embryology. 4th edition. (Figure 14-14). Philadelphia: Churchill Livingstone/Elsevier; 2009; with permission.)

Development of the Enteric Nervous System

Neural crest cells are the source of the enteric nervous system (ENS). The vagal neural crest supplies ganglia to the intestine, and its innervation is completed by week 13 of development. Disturbances of this process can result in genetic abnormalities, such as Hirschsprung disease and intestinal neuronal dysplasia.

ANATOMY

Macroscopic Features

At the most basic level, the small intestine is a 6- to 7-m-long hollow tube that begins at the pylorus and ends at the ileocecal valve. The most proximal portion of the intestine is the duodenum, which is traditionally divided into 4 sections (**Fig. 2**). The duodenum starts at the pylorus with the duodenal bulb; superficially this corresponds to just above the level of the umbilicus. The first part of the duodenum is the only portion that is not retroperitoneal and is instead connected to the liver by a part of the lesser omentum called the hepatoduodenal ligament.[10] The duodenum then quickly travels into the retroperitoneal space and descends as it sweeps around the head of the pancreas. The descending portion of the duodenum is the site of the major and minor duodenal papilla. The major duodenal papilla serves as the common entrance for the bile and pancreatic ducts, whereas the minor duodenal papilla is the entrance for the accessory pancreatic ducts. The duodenum then returns to the peritoneal cavity at the level of the L2 vertebra, where it is fixed to the retroperitoneum by a suspensory ligament called the ligament of Treitz, marking the transition from duodenum to jejunum.

The jejunum resides primarily in the left upper quadrant of the abdomen, is approximately 2.5 m in length, and is suspended in the peritoneal cavity by a thin mesentery attached to the posterior abdominal wall, which allows for relatively free movement.[11] Examination of the luminal surface of the jejunum reveals plicae circulares, which represent circular mucosal and submucosa folds that serve to increase surface area. Plicae

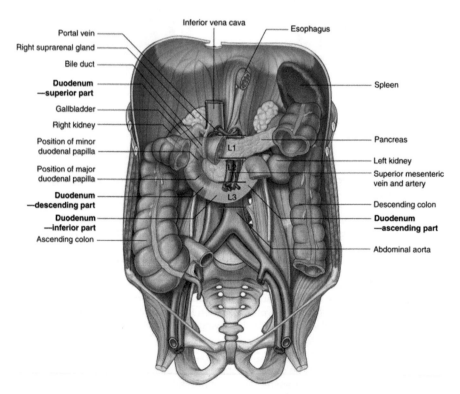

Fig. 2. Anatomy of the duodenum. (*From* Drake RL, Vogl AW, Mitchell AWM. Gray's anatomy for students. Philadelphia: Churchill-Livingstone; 2015; with permission)

circulares are particularly numerous in the proximal jejunum but also exist in the duodenum and decrease as one moves distally in the small bowel and are totally absent by the terminal ileum.[12] Lymphoid follicles can be visualized in the small intestine, particularly in children. They are most numerous in the ileum and are called Peyer patches.

The jejunum transitions to the ileum without an anatomic delineation and is primarily found in the right lower abdomen and pelvis. The jejunum is distinguished from the ileum by its thicker lumen and more prominent mucosal folds. The small bowel ends at the ileocecal valve, which is composed of 2 semilunar lips that protrude into the cecum and serve as a barrier to retrograde flow of colonic contents into the small intestine. The function of the valve relies on the angulation between the ileum and cecum, which is created by the superior and inferior ileocecal ligaments.[13] The mesentery is a double-layered fold of peritoneum with fat, blood vessels and the lymphatic system residing within these layers. Its superior attachment is at the duodenal-jejunum junction, and its posterior attachment is near the ileocecal junction at the upper border of the right sacro-iliac joint.[14]

Histology

The small intestine is composed of 4 layers: mucosa, submucosa, muscularis propria, and adventitia (serosa).

Mucosa

The lumen-facing surface of the small intestine is lined by the mucosa, which is composed of 3 distinct layers: epithelium, laminal propria, and muscularis mucosae. The predominant cell type of the epithelium is absorptive cells called enterocytes. Each enterocyte has approximately 3000 microvilli at its luminal surface, which appear as a striated brush border on the surface of the villi. The villi, microvilli and plicae circulares together increase the absorptive surface of the small intestine by 600-fold.

The epithelial cells lining the lumen are organized in a crypt-villi axis and are constantly proliferating and differentiating. Fueling this proliferation are intestinal stem cells located in the crypt base.[15] As the cells differentiate, they migrate in a vertical direction to the apical portion of the villus. These cells differentiate into 1 of 7 different cell types (absorptive enterocytes, enteroendocrine cells, Paneth cell, goblet cells, tuft cell, cup cells, and M cells). These terminally differentiated cells serve many roles, as outlined in **Table 2**.

Adjacent epithelial cells are held together at their apical pole by tight junctions called zona occludens. These complexes serve as an important regulator of transcellular transportation.[16]

The lamina propria provides a base of connective tissue that supports the epithelium. Lymphocytes and mast cells are found within the lamina propria and represent the largest mass of immunoprotective tissue in the body.[17]

Below the lamina propria is the muscularis mucosa, a thin layer of smooth muscle that plays a minor role in intestinal peristalsis.

Submucosa

The submucosa is a connective tissue layer composed of fibroblasts and mast cells. Within the submucosa is a dense network of arteries and lymphatic tissue that aid the small intestine in its absorptive role. Specialized cells in the submucosal layer of the duodenum secrete mucus and bicarbonate to help neutralize acidic gastric contents. In the submucosa is a collection of nerves and ganglion called the submucosal plexus that communicates with the myenteric plexus to coordinate peristalsis.

Table 2
Intestinal epithelial cell types and function

Cell	Function	Structure	Location
Enterocytes	The main absorptive cell of the small intestine	Tall columnar cells with microvilli on the apical side; bound to each other by junction complexes	Predominant cell type of the epithelium
Paneth cells	Secrete lyzosyme and defensing, which serve as a defense against bacteria and may regulate intestinal flora	Large, pyramidal cells with eosinophilic granules at their apical end that contain lysozyme and other glycoproteins	Base of crypts of Lieberkuhn
Enteroendocrine cells	Locally regulate intestinal activity by secreting hormones (CCK, secretin, GIP) into the capillaries	Granules are closer at the basal rather than apical end of the cell	Primarily located in the crypts but can be found at other locations within the epithelium
Goblet cells	Mucin secreting cells that serve a cytoprotective role and lubricating role in the GI tract	Goblet shaped with large granules located apically in the cell	Located throughout the small intestine, greater concentration in the ileum than the jejunum
Tuft cells	Serve a role in chemoreception and potentially parasitic defense	Have an apical bundle of microfilaments connected to a long microvilli that protrudes into the lumen	A rare cell type comprising 0.4% of intestinal epithelium
Cup cells	The apical end is broad and tapers toward the base	No current known function	Limited to the ileum
M cells	Antigen sampling cells that endocytose bacteria and viruses from the lumen to Peyer patch	Epithelial cells that lack a brush border and have many apical endocytic vesicles	Overlie Peyer patch

From Yamada T, Alpers DH. Textbook of gastroenterology. Philadelphia: Lippincott Williams & Wilkins; 2003.

Muscularis propria
The muscularis propria is primarily responsible for peristalsis of the small intestine. It consists of 2 layers of muscle: the inner circular layer and the outer longitudinal layer. Between these layers is the myenteric (also known as Auerbach) plexus composed of parasympathetic and postganglionic sympathetic fibers. The myenteric nerve plexus is essential for coordinating peristalsis.

Adventitia (serosa)
The serosa is composed of a thin lining of mesothelial cells with an underlying loose connective tissue structure.

Circulation

Oxygenated blood to the duodenum, jejunum, and ileum arrives primarily from the superior mesenteric artery (SMA). The duodenum is the exception with blood supplied not only from the SMA but also from branches of the gastroduodenal artery, which itself is a branch of the hepatic artery. Venous drainage is handled primarily by the superior mesenteric vein, which later joins the splenic vein to form the portal system.

Lymphatic System

The lymphatic system of the small intestine is composed of small lymphatic capillaries called the villus lacteals that reside within small intestinal villi. These lymphatic channels drain into the mesenteric lymph nodes located along the SMA.

NEURONAL INNERVATION
Extrinsic Innervation

The smooth muscle and secretory cells of the small intestine come under the dual influence of the sympathetic and parasympathetic divisions of the autonomic nervous system (ANS). The dorsal nucleus of the vagus nerve, located in the brain stem, sends long preganglionic axons to the postganglionic effector neurons in the small intestine wall (see later discussion). Acetylcholine is the primary chemical mediator and is generally stimulatory in nature. Sympathetic innervation to the small intestine begins with cells in the intermediolateral cell column of the thoracic spinal cord (thoracic segments T5-T11). Preganglionic fibers pass without interruption through the sympathetic trunk, form the greater and lesser splanchnic nerves, and then terminate in the celiac ganglion and superior mesenteric ganglion (located within their respective plexuses). Norepinephrine, the primary neurotransmitter (NT) in the postganglionic neurons, is typically inhibitory in nature. Physiologically, extrinsic innervation by the ANS modulates small intestine activity, although its presence is not absolutely required, because small intestine motor activity persists despite vagotomy or splanchnicectomy.[18] The ability of the small intestine to function autonomously is due in large part to the ENS (described in later discussion).

Intrinsic Innervation

The ENS consists of nerve cell bodies and their processes embedded in the wall of the gut. It originates from neural crest cells, and when fully developed contains 200 to 600 million neurons.[19] The ENS is intimately involved in complex issues of small intestine motility, secretion, and blood flow. Collections of these nerve cell bodies form the enteric ganglia, which are connected by an extensive network of nerve cell processes to form 2 major ganglionated plexuses.[20] The myenteric plexus lies between the external longitudinal and inner circular muscle layer of the GI tract.[21] It forms a continuous network and extends from the upper esophagus to the internal anal sphincter. The myenteric plexus primarily provides motor innervation to the 2 muscle layers and secretomotor innervation to the mucosa. Each ganglion in the myenteric plexus may contain up to 200 cells. The ganglia are connected to each other by small bands of nerve fibers called internodal strands, which branch off and innervate the circular smooth muscle. Bundles of nerve fibers also run through the circular muscle layer to connect the myenteric plexus with the submucosal and mucosal plexuses. The submucosal plexus lies between the inner circular muscle layer and the mucosa and is primarily found in the small and large intestine. Although ganglia are occasionally found in the esophagus and stomach, the submucosal plexus does not form an extensive network here. Neurons in the submucosal plexus innervate secretory cells, endocrine cells, and blood vessels in the mucosa and submucosa. In addition, intrinsic sensory neurons, also called primary afferent neurons (IPANs), project from the submucosal plexus to the myenteric plexus (IPANs are also found in the myenteric plexus).

The myenteric plexus and the submucosal plexus are the major components of the ENS; however, several small nonganglionated plexuses also play a role in small intestine motility, including the longitudinal muscle plexus, the circular muscle plexus, the mucosal plexus, the plexus of the muscularis mucosa, and the perivascular plexus.

As in all nervous systems involved in sensory-motor function, neurons in the ENS can be classified into 3 general classes of neurons. The first class is IPANs, which are sensitive to chemical and mechanical stimuli. IPANs are present in both the submucosal and the myenteric plexuses, respond to chemical stimuli in the gut lumen, and stretch and distend the gut lumen and mucosa. IPANs form multiple connections with circular and longitudinal motor neurons, other sensory neurons, and interneurons, and these pathways both ascend and descend with the GI tract. The second class is interneurons, which are interposed between sensory neurons and motor neurons, and form a network to link interneurons to one another. Both ascending and descending pathways are present. Interneurons play a vital role in amplifying and distributing signals throughout the gut and are involved in motor, secretory, and vasomotor functions. The third class is motor neurons. These motor neurons act on different effector cells, including smooth muscle, blood vessels, pacemaker cells of the gut, mucosal glands, and mucosal cells and can be either excitatory in nature or inhibitory.

PHYSIOLOGY
Signaling Within the Small Intestine (Neurotransmitters and Hormones)

Neurotransmitters
More than 35 different NTs have been identified in enteric neurons. Individual neurons of the ENS generally contain several NTs, although a single predominant NT typically characterizes its mode of action.[22] Vasoconstrictor neurons in the submucosal plexus contain a predominance of norepinephrine, while inhibitory motor neurons in the myenteric plexus contain predominantly vasoactive intestinal polypeptide (VIP), nitric oxide (NO), adenosine triphosphate (ATP), and pituitary activating cyclic AMP peptide. In general, acetylcholine, substance P, and tachykinins are the major excitatory NTs in the GI tract, whereas NO and VIP are the major inhibitory NTs. Serotonin plays a critical role in gut motor, sensory, and secretory function and is found in a variety of neurons, especially the interneurons.

Hormones
A variety of growth factors and hormones are important during early development, although their effects on small intestine motility in adults have not been well studied. Insulin-like growth factor and epidermal growth factor both play a trophic role in small intestine mucosal growth and viability.[23] Reduced or absent levels of glucocorticoids, which can occur after adrenal injury, may lead to mucosal atrophy and villous disorganization.

Motility

Smooth muscle
The smooth muscle of the small intestine exhibits continuous fluctuations in membrane potential; these are called slow waves and occur with a frequency of approximately 11 to 12 times per minute (a lower frequency is observed in the terminal ileum, approximately 7–8/min). Studies in mice deficient in the Kit tyrosinase-kinase receptor have identified the interstitial cells of Cajal (ICC) as being responsible for

generating the slow wave.[24] In the proper neurohumoral setting (neural, endocrine, and/or paracrine modulation), action potentials are elicited in the form of a spike burst. This spike burst results in a smooth muscle contraction, which spreads circumferentially first and then spreads along the small intestine in an aboral direction. Clinically, several disorders can affect smooth muscle cells of the small intestine, leading to disturbances in motility. The most common of these disorders include connective tissue disorders (eg, scleroderma); infiltrative disorders (ie, amyloid, lymphoma, sarcoid); long-term steroid use; and inherited conditions (eg, chronic intestinal pseudoobstruction of the myopathic type).

Interstitial cells of Cajal

The ICC are small (20 μm), specialized cells located in the muscle layers of the GI tract. These cells are considered to be the pacemaker cells of the gut. ICC generate spontaneous, rhythmic, slow waves of depolarization in intestinal smooth muscle and are involved in the coordination of the electromechanical activity of the gut. ICC are not identical throughout the GI tract, but vary from region to region. In the stomach, ICC have a slow-wave rhythm of 3 cpm, whereas in the small intestine it is approximately 11 to 12 cpm. ICC can be identified by staining for the tyrosine-kinase receptor, c-kit. Clinically, loss of ICC leads to intestinal pseudo-obstruction.

Peristalsis

Small intestine motility can be measured in several different ways (ie, fluoroscopy, wireless pH capsule, scintigraphy); however, small intestine manometry is thought to provide the most meaningful physiologic information. That said, it is important to recognize that intraluminal manometry detects pressure waves generated by the circular muscle layer. Reliable in vivo information on tonic smooth muscle activity and the longitudinal muscle layer is lacking. Similar to the stomach, the migrating motor complex (MMC) plays a critical role in small bowel motility. Using intraluminal motility catheters, the MMC is observed in the fasting state, and a wave of contraction (phase III of the MMC) can pass through the small intestine every 80 to 120 minutes (phase I is a period of quiescence; phase II is a period of chaotic activity).[25] Phase III of the MMC typically lasts 5 to 7 minutes with a mean amplitude of 30 mm Hg and a velocity of 5 to 10 cm/min in the proximal small intestine.[26] The MMC is generally initiated in the gastroduodenal region; however, the presence of multiple small intestine pacemakers allows for the initiation of an MMC even when the small intestine has been disrupted surgically. When food is ingested, the MMC is interrupted and an irregular pattern of contractility develops. The interruption slows small intestine transit time, increases mucosal contact time, and thus allows for more efficient absorption of nutrients, electrolytes, and water. Distention of the small intestine lumen, change in pH, and hyperosmolar solutions all slow small intestine transit time as well. Thus, small intestine transit is most rapid during phase III of the MMC, while absorption is greatest during phase I. Absence of the MMC and absence of a phase III during the MMC (with a minimum of 8 hours of recording) are considered markers of severe enteric neuromuscular dysfunction.[27]

Digestion and Absorption

Most chemical digestion takes place in the small intestine; however, the act of digestion relies on a complex interplay that involves nearly every component of the GI tract.

Lipids

Dietary lipids are primarily absorbed by the upper two-thirds of the jejunum. Before absorption, they undergo several digestive steps due to their insoluble nature in water.

A comprehensive review of this complex process is beyond the scope of this article, although a brief outline follows.

Lipid digestion starts with the breakdown of triglycerides, which involves the removal of fatty acids from their glycerol backbones by lipase. Although this begins in the stomach, most lipolysis occurs in the small intestine. Pancreatic lipase enters the small bowel via the pancreatic duct and requires a nearly neutral pH created by secretion of bicarbonate from the pancreas and biliary tree. Pancreatic lipase binds to the mucosal brush border, which aids in the rapid absorption of fatty acids and other products of lipid digestion. Bile salts serve to emulsify triglycerides, increasing access of triglycerides to lipase. The transport of fatty acids is partially dependent on the formation of micelles with bile salts. The micelles help fatty acids cross the unstirred water layer and gain access to the small intestine brush border for rapid absorption. Absorption into enterocytes was long thought to be a passive process; however, several fatty acid binding proteins that serve as carrier-mediated transporters have been recently discovered (called fatty acid transport proteins) demonstrating that this is a more active process.[28] Once inside enterocytes fatty acids bind to fatty acid binding proteins that are concentrated in villus cells. These proteins transfer the fatty acids across the cytoplasm to the endoplasmic reticulum where they are resynthesized.

Carbohydrates

Digestion of carbohydrates is a multistep process with many of the steps dependent on the small bowel and its unique properties. The first step of carbohydrate digestion involves hydrolysis of starch in the intestinal lumen. Although salivary amylase plays a role, it is minor compared with the role of pancreatic amylase.[29] Pancreatic amylase initiates the digestion of starch by cleaving α-(1,4)-glycosidic linkages of the starch molecule, resulting in the production of maltose and maltotriose as well as oligosaccharides that remain as a result of amylase's inability to cleave α-(1,6)-bonds. This process is completed by the time luminal contents reach the proximal jejunum.[30]

The resulting maltose, maltotriose, and disaccharides undergo further hydrolysis aided by one of several carbohydrases located in the apical membrane of duodenal and jejunal enterocytes (**Table 3**). The oligosaccharides produced earlier during luminal digestion are next hydrolyzed to glucose by α-dextrinase. The resulting monosaccharides can then be transported across the apical membrane.

The monosaccharides, primarily glucose, galactose, and fructose, are then transported across the apical and basolateral membranes of the enterocytes. Transportation is accomplished using carrier-mediated transporters located in the brush border of enterocytes. Glucose and galactose are transported by a sodium cotransporter called the sodium-glucose cotransporter (SGLT1). This process is fueled by a Na, K, ATPase pump, which generates a low intracellular Na^+ concentration, thereby fueling cotransport of glucose via SGLT1.[31] Glucose and galactose then exit the basolateral

Table 3		
Major brush border carbohydrases		
Substrate	**Enzyme**	**End Product**
α-1,4-Linked oligosaccharides	Maltase	Glucose
Lactose	Lactase	Glucose and galactose
Sucrose	Sucrase	Glucose and fructose
α-Limit dextrins	Isomaltase	Glucose

membrane via facilitated diffusion driven by a glucose transporter called GLUT2. Fructose is handled in a similar manner with the exception that it enters into the enterocyte mediated by GLUT5 via facilitated diffusion rather than a cotransporter system.

Protein

Proteins are degraded into small peptides and amino acids before absorption. This process begins in the stomach through the action of pepsins. By the time the digested contents reach the small intestine, the proteins have been broken down to polypeptides and amino acids. Because of pepsins' activity at acidic pH, it is no longer active by the time it reaches the small bowel. In the small bowel, pancreatic proteolytic enzymes continue the process of protein digestion. Proteolytic enzymes, including trypsin and chymotrypsin, are secreted by the pancreas and cleave proteins into oligopeptides and amino acids (**Table 4**). Pancreatic proteolytic enzymes are not released in an active form from the pancreas and therefore must be activated once within the intestinal lumen. Enterokinase serves this important role of activating trypsinogen to trypsin. This enterokinase functions by removing the hexapeptide NH_2-terminal end from trypsinogen to produce trypsin. Trypsin is then able to activate other proteases including trypsinogen. The pancreatic proteolytic enzymes together cleave proteins into smaller and smaller peptides. There are a range of peptidases present in the brush border and in the cytoplasm of enterocytes that continue oligopeptide digestion, Explaining why most protein end products that reach the portal circulation are amino acids and not oligopeptides.

Protein end products are absorbed by enterocytes as dipeptides, tripeptides, and amino acids. The transport of dipeptides and tripeptides appears to rely on a single transporter called Pept-1. This transporter relies on an electrochemical H^+ gradient as its driving force.[32] Transport of amino acids across the villus of enterocytes relies on several distinct carrier-mediated active and facilitated transport proteins. Transport of peptides and amino acids across the basolateral membrane relies on various mechanisms involving both active and facilitated transport.

Folate

Folate is absorbed in the duodenum and upper jejunum. Dietary folate is hydrolyzed by glutamate carboxypeptidase II at the brush border and is actively transported into the enterocyte by the reduced folate carrier where it enters the portal circulation.

Cobalamin (Vitamin B12)

Cobalamin reaches the small intestine after binding to the R protein (haptocorrin) in the gastric lumen. In the small intestine where pH is higher than the gastric environment, intrinsic factor (IF) has a higher affinity for cobalamin than R protein. R protein is

Table 4	
Pancreatic proteolytic enzymes and their function	
Proteolytic Enzyme	**Function**
Trypsin	Cleaves bonds at lysine or arginine; cleaves pancreatic proenzymes
Elastase	Cleaves bond at aliphatic amino acid
Chymotrypsin	Cleaves bonds at aromatic or neutral amino acids
Carboxypeptidase A	Cleaves aromatic amino acids at terminal ends of peptides
Carboxypeptidase B	Cleaves arginine or lysine from terminal ends of peptides

From Feldman M, Friedman LS, Sleisenger MH. Sleisenger & Fordtran's gastrointestinal and liver disease: pathophysiology, diagnosis, management. Philadelphia: Saunders; 2002.

hydrolyzed by various pancreatic enzymes, leaving cobalamin to bind with IF, which is secreted by parietal cells. The cobalamin-IF complex passes to the terminal ileum, where it binds to receptors on the ileal surface called cubulin-amnionless (AML).[33] The cobalamin-IF-AML complex is now able to enter the enterocyte.

Fat-soluble vitamins

Vitamins A, D, and E are absorbed passively in the small intestine. Vitamin K is absorbed in the small intestine as well. Vitamin K_1, which is derived primarily from plants, is dependent on luminal bile salts and carrier-mediated diffusion. Vitamin K_2, which is produced by gut bacteria, is able to be absorbed passively.

Water

The small intestine plays a primary role in the absorption of the approximately 9.0 L of water delivered to the GI tract daily. The small bowel is responsible for absorbing 7 to 8 L of this water (60%–80% efficient) with the colon absorbing the remainder, with the exception of the 100 to 200 mL that is excreted in the stool. The mechanism of water absorption has not been well explained to date. It is thought to occur primarily as a function of electrolyte and osmotic gradients that result from the transport of electrolytes. In addition to an osmotic driving force, aquaporins have been discovered in intestinal membranes. Despite their discovery, their role is unclear.

REFERENCES

1. Zorn AM, Wells JM. Vertebrate endoderm development and organ formation. Annu Rev Cell Dev Biol 2009;25:221–51.
2. Beddington RS, Smith JC. Control of vertebrate gastrulation: inducing signals and responding genes. Curr Opin Genet Dev 1993;3:655–61.
3. Beck F. The role of Cdx genes in the mammalian gut. Gut 2004;53:1394–6.
4. Schoenwolf GC, Larsen WJ. Larsen's human embryology. Philadelphia: Churchill Livingstone/Elsevier; 2009. p. 82–107.
5. Grand RJ, Watkins JB, Torti FM. Development of intestinal tract. Gastroenterology 1976;70:1271–6.
6. Spence JR, Lauf R, Shroyer NF. Vertebrate intestinal endoderm development. Dev Dyn 2011;240:501–20.
7. Reya T, Clevers H. Wnt signaling in stem cells and cancer. Nature 2005;434:843.
8. Fre S, Huyghe M, Mourikis P, et al. Notch signals control the fate of immature progenitor cells in the intestine. Nature 2005;435:964.
9. Madison BB, Braunstein K, Kuizon E, et al. Epithelial hedgehog signals patter the intestinal crypt-villus axis. Development 2005;132:279.
10. Shepherd R. Grays anatomy. London: Stanhope Books; 2014.
11. Feldman M, Friedman LS, Sleisenger MH. Sleisenger & Fordtran's gastrointestinal and liver disease: pathophysiology, diagnosis, management. Philadelphia: Saunders; 2002.
12. Yamada T, Alpers DH. Textbook of gastroenterology. Philadelphia: Lippincott Williams & Wilkins; 2003.
13. Kumar D, Phillips SF. The contribution of external ligamentous attachments to function of the ileocecal junction. Dis Colon Rectum 1987;30:410–6.
14. Gray H, Pick TP, Howden R. Gray's anatomy. East Molesey (UK): Senate; 2003.
15. Potten CS, Gandara R, Mahida YR, et al. The stem cells of small intestinal crypts: where are they? Cell Prolif 2009;42:731–50.
16. Anderson JM, Van Itallie CM. Tight junctions and the molecular basis for regulation of paracellular permeability. Am J Physiol 1995;269:G467–75.

17. Floch NR. Netter's gastroenterology. Philadelphia: Elsevier Saunders; 2005.

18. Kunze WA, Furness JB. The enteric nervous system and regulation of intestinal motility. Annu Rev Physiol 1999;61:117–42.

19. Furness JB. The enteric nervous system. Oxford (UK): Blackwell; 2006.

20. Gershon MD. The enteric nervous system. Annu Rev Neurosci 1981;4:227–72.

21. Sternini C. Structural and chemical organization of the myenteric plexus. Annu Rev Physiol 1988;50:81–93.

22. Furness JB, Costa M, Gibbins I, et al. Neurochemically similar myenteric and submucous neurons directly traced to the mucosa of the small intestine. Cell Tissue Res 1985;241:155–63.

23. Drozdowski L, Thomson AB. Intestinal hormones and growth factors: effects on the small intestine. World J Gastroenterol 2009;15:385–406.

24. Huizinga JD, Thuneberg L, Kluppel M, et al. The W/kit gene required for interstitial cells of Cajal and intestinal pacemaker activity. Nature 1995;373:347–9.

25. Vantrappen G, Janssens J, Hellemans J, et al. The interdigestive motor complex of normal subjects and patients with bacterial overgrowth of the small intestine. J Clin Invest 1977;59:1158–66.

26. Kellow JE, Borody S, Phillips S, et al. Human interdigestive motility: variations in patterns from esophagus to colon. Gastroenterology 1986;91:386–95.

27. Malagelada JR, Stanghellini V. Manometric evaluation of functional upper gut symptoms. Gastroenterology 1985;88:1223–31.

28. Stahl A, Gimeno RE, Tartaglia LA, et al. Fatty acid transport proteins: a current view of a growing family. Trends Endocrinol Metab 2001;12:266–73.

29. Guzman-Maldonado H, Paredes-Lopez O. Amylolytic enzymes and products derived from starch: a review. Crit Rev Food Sci Nutr 1995;35:373–403.

30. Layer P, Zinsmeister AR, DiMagno EP. Effects of decreasing intraluminal amylase activity on starch digestion and postprandial gastrointestinal function in humans. Gastroenterology 1986;91:41.

31. Wright EM, Hirayama BA, Loo DF. Active sugar transport in health and disease. J Intern Med 2007;261:32–43.

32. Adibi SA. The oligopeptide transporter (Pept-1) in human intestine: biology and function. Gastroenterology 1997;113:332–40.

33. Christensen EI, Birn H. Megalin and cubilin: multifunctional endocytic receptors. Nat Rev Mol Cell Biol 2002;3:256–66.

Video Capsule Endoscopy
Technology, Reading, and Troubleshooting

Jodie A. Barkin, MD*, Jamie S. Barkin, MD, MACG, MACP, AGAF, FASGE

KEYWORDS

- Video capsule endoscopy • Obscure gastrointestinal bleeding
- Small bowel bleeding • Technology • Reading • Contraindications • Preparation

KEY POINTS

- Video capsule endoscopy can be performed in inpatients and outpatients, requires appropriate bowel preparation before the study, and can be administered via oral swallowing or endoscopic device placement into the small bowel based on outlined patient-dependent factors.
- Current commercially available video capsule endoscopy systems were reviewed and compared for individual features and attributes.
- Reading a video capsule endoscopy study should be done in a systematic manner, including identification of anatomic landmarks, calculation of small bowel transit time, objective assessment of the quality of bowel preparation, and detailed description of any abnormal findings.
- There are multiple contraindications and risks to video capsule endoscopy, which need to be carefully weighed with an appropriate informed consent process between patient and provider.

INTRODUCTION

Video capsule endoscopy (VCE) has completed the endoscopic visualization of the entire luminal gastrointestinal tract. It has taken us on a "fantastic voyage," which is improving with each technical advance. Knowledge of its indications, preparation, and contraindications will allow us to apply this endoscopic technology in a precise and accurate manner. This article focuses on preparation for VCE, currently available VCE technology, how to read a VCE study, and risks and contraindications to VCE.

Disclosure Statement: The authors have nothing to disclose.
Division of Gastroenterology, Department of Medicine, Leonard M. Miller School of Medicine, University of Miami, 1120 North West 14th Street, Clinical Research Building, Suite 1116 (D-49), Miami, FL 33136, USA
* Corresponding author.
E-mail address: jabarkin@med.miami.edu

Gastrointest Endoscopy Clin N Am 27 (2017) 15–27
http://dx.doi.org/10.1016/j.giec.2016.08.002
1052-5157/17/© 2016 Elsevier Inc. All rights reserved.

giendo.theclinics.com

VIDEO CAPSULE ENDOSCOPY: PREPARATION, ADMINISTRATION, AND COMPLETION

VCE can be performed in both inpatients and outpatients. Patients are generally recommended to remain on a clear liquid diet the day before VCE administration. A 2009 meta-analysis of 12 studies by Rokkas and colleagues[1] demonstrated the importance of bowel preparation in comparison to clear liquid diet to improve small bowel visualization quality and to increase the diagnostic yield of VCE examinations. Bowel preparation with 2 L of polyethylene glycol is common and provides relatively comparable preparation quality and diagnostic yield to a 4-L polyethylene glycol preparation.[2] Newer low-volume bowel preparations using MoviPrep or Pico-Salax have also been suggested to have comparable efficacy.[3] Simethicone may be administered before VCE to reduce the presence of bubbles in the small bowel.

Narcotics and other medications such as anticholinergics and antihistamines, which may cause gastroparesis, should be stopped if possible 2 to 3 days before VCE administration. Alternatively, patients can receive either metoclopramide 10 mg 3 times daily before meals or erythromycin 250 mg every 8 hours for 2 to 3 days before VCE administration; however, endoscopic placement may be needed given potential medication-induced gastroparesis. Cessation or dose reduction of anticoagulants, including warfarin or the novel anticoagulants, is not recommended before VCE administration, and diagnostic yield of VCE may actually be increased if bleeding is provoked during the study.[4,5]

VCE administration can be performed using 2 methods: swallowing the VCE by mouth or endoscopic deployment of the VCE into the small bowel. Oral VCE administration is more common, with obvious benefit by foregoing an additional invasive procedure with all associated risks, and marked cost savings of the endoscopic procedure and sedation. Following oral VCE administration, patients may ingest clear liquids 2 hours later and may have a light meal 4 hours after VCE administration. Failure to reach the cecum during the recorded time resulting in an incomplete study is estimated to occur in up to 19% to 27% of patients undergoing VCE via oral administration.[6,7] A portion of these patients may be able to achieve a complete VCE study with endoscopic deployment.

Endoscopic deployment should be considered in patients with known or anticipated difficulty of the VCE passing from the mouth to the small bowel in a safe and timely manner to enable maximal small bowel mucosal visualization and to ensure a complete capsule study. These factors include patients with known inability to swallow (oropharyngeal, esophageal, or both, such as after a cerebrovascular accident, musculoskeletal disorders, poor nutrition with undiagnosed dysphagia, and known dysphagia), gastroparesis, opioid usage with delayed gastric transit, hospitalized patients, especially those who are bedbound and patients in the intensive care unit, and those with prior capsule failing to reach the cecum. Although increasingly common, patients with prior bariatric or gastric surgery may satisfactorily undergo oral VCE administration with similar completion rates to the general population.[8]

Lack of physical activity such as in patients who are on strict bed rest is significantly associated with an incomplete VCE study compared with those who are ambulatory or with mild bed rest.[9] Real-time viewer features found on certain capsule devices may assist the endoscopist in the placement of the capsule device into the duodenum in particularly challenging cases.[10] Despite endoscopic placement, there still remains a subset of patients in whom VCE may be incomplete, perhaps due to underlying structural or motility disorders.[11] Importantly, endoscopic sedation with propofol on the same day as VCE increases small bowel transit time (SBTT), but does not affect VCE completion rates.[12]

Prokinetic agents may be used to promote VCE exit from the stomach into the small bowel in patients undergoing oral capsule administration and should be considered in inpatients or those with limited mobility. A dose of metoclopramide 10 mg can be given either by endoscopy unit protocol after oral VCE administration or by examination of a real-time viewer at a set point such as 30 to 60 minutes after oral VCE administration to determine if the VCE remains in the stomach. Although metoclopramide is the most common prokinetic used, erythromycin and domperidone administration with VCE may result in a slightly higher completion rate to the cecum for the study, but no tangible effect on diagnostic yield of the VCE study.[13,14]

VIDEO CAPSULE ENDOSCOPY SYSTEMS

There are 5 commercially available VCE systems, with corresponding individual software programs for reading the recorded study images. Each system has unique features, which are aimed to address the inability to control VCE movement, to increase completion rate of a VCE study, and ultimately improve diagnostic yield (**Table 1**).

PillCam SB1, SB2, SB3

The PillCam (Given Imaging Ltd, Yoqneam, Israel) was the first commercially available VCE system approved in the United States in 2001. Since then, there have been 3 generations of the PillCam, with most institutions currently using the SB2 or SB3 capsule systems. The PillCam SB2 system is approximately 26 × 11 mm in size and 3.45 g in weight, whereas the PillCam SB3 system is the same size but weighs 1.9 g. The SB2 captures 2 frames per second, using a complementary metal-oxide semiconductor for image capturing, and 6 white light–emitting diodes for illumination. Increasing frame rate from 2 to 4 frames per second has been examined in a study of 89 patients comparing the PillCam SB2 and the PillCam SB2$_4$ systems, which showed no significant clinical impact from the increased frame rate and increased overall reading times, but may have additional benefit in some selected situations to better visualize

Table 1
Comparison of video capsule endoscopes for small bowel imaging

	PillCam SB3	EndoCapsule 10	CapsoCam SV1	MiroCam	OMOM
Manufacturer	Given Imaging	Olympus	CapsoVision	IntroMedic	Jianshan
Length (mm)	26	26	31	24.5	28
Diameter (mm)	11	11	11	10.8	13
Weight (g)	1.9	3.3	4	3.25	
Type of image sensor	CMOS	CCD	CMOS	CMOS	CMOS
Frame rate (per second)	2–6 (adaptive frame rate)	2	20 (5 per camera) first 2 h then 12 (3 per camera) thereafter	3	2
Number of cameras	1	1	4	1	1
Field of view (°)	156	160	360	170	140
Battery life (h)	12	12	15	12	8

Abbreviations: CCD, charge coupled device; CMOS, complementary metal-oxide semiconductor.

a lesion.[15] The newer generation SB3 system has a 156° field of view, and an adaptive frame rate of 2 to 6 frames per second. More pictures are taken per second when the capsule is moving quicker and less as the capsule is moving slower, which may reduce duplication of images and therefore reading time. The original PillCam SB2 system has an 8-hour battery life, whereas newer models including the SB3 have increased battery life up to 12 to 15 hours. Images are transmitted from the device to a receiver band using radiofrequency, and the SB2 and SB3 models also have a small screen on the recorder for real-time viewing.[16–19]

The accompanying PillCam Rapid Reader software includes the "Quick View" mode, which is an informatics algorithm that can shorten reading time while also attempting to increase diagnostic yield.[20] Furthermore, the Rapid Reader viewing software also enables reviewer-controlled playback speed and number of images (1, 2, 4, or collage; although the collage mode is not intended for reading). There is an accompanying digital image atlas, and the "Suspected Blood Indicator" feature by which certain images with a cluster of red-colored pixels that may indicate blood or a lesion are highlighted.[19,21] The "Suspected Blood Indicator" feature may further alert a reader to an area of concern. However, its utility in identifying lesions is limited, and therefore, it should not be relied on as a reading tool.

Endocapsule

The Endocapsule (Olympus Corporation, Tokyo, Japan) was the second commercially available VCE system, entering the market in 2008. The newest generation of this system, the Endocapsule 10, captures 2 frames per second of a 160° field of view and is of similar size at 26 × 11 mm and weight to other systems. This system uses 6 white light–emitting diodes for illumination, a charge coupled device for image sensing, and radiofrequency for transmitting images from the device to the receiver. It has up to a 12-hour battery life, and a real-time viewer on the receiver. The newest version of accompanying reading software has a 3-dimensional (3D) tracking function designed to track capsule progress through the small intestine and denotes this on each thumbnail picture, and automatic features to detect and remove poor quality images that would be unable to be read to expedite reviewing time. Furthermore, the reading software is equipped with an overview function, and both an express-selected mode and an auto-speed-adjusted mode to reduce redundant images, with the goal of decreased reading times while still maintaining diagnostic yield.[22–25]

CapsoCam

The CapsoCam SV-1 (CapsoVision Inc, Saratoga, CA, USA) system entered international markets beginning in 2012 and was approved in the United States in 2016. It incorporates 4 laterally placed cameras facing the digestive wall offering 360° of viewing, without forward and backward viewing. Five frames per camera per second of images (20 frames/s in total) are taken in the first 2 hours of recording and then 3 frames per camera per second (12 frames/s in total) are taken thereafter. It has a maximal recording time of 15 total hours based on battery life. This specific capsule is 11 × 31 mm in size and 4 g in weight, has a complementary metal-oxide semiconductor in each camera, and uses 16 white light–emitting diodes, with an auto illumination controller to optimize light settings. It uses "Smart Motion Sense" technology to only activate the cameras when the capsule is moving, thereby reducing redundant images and saving battery life. Since 2012, there have been 2 subsequent generations of CapsoCam, although SV-1 remains the only US Food and Drug Administration–approved CapsoCam system in the United States currently. Of note, the CapsoCam stores images on board the device itself and does not transmit images to any external recording device. Therefore, patients must collect the capsule using a collecting pan and a magnetic wand and then return the device for downloading. Reading is performed using a 4-image viewer on the software with frequency of approximately 8 frames per second (total speed 32 frames/s based on 4 simultaneous image viewing). Furthermore, visualization of the ampulla has been reported at 71% in one series, which may positively impact diagnostic yield in the future.[16,26,27]

MiroCam

The MiroCam capsule (IntroMedic, Seoul, Korea) captures 3 frames per second, with a 170° field of view, using a complementary oxide silicone chip for imaging, and measures 10.8 × 24.5 mm in size, and approximately 3.25 g in weight. This device does not use radiofrequency transmission and instead transmits recorded images using electric-field propagation by using 2 gold plates on the capsule surface in order to transmit low-voltage signals through the human body and to record electrodes attached to the skin, thereby decreasing power requirements and increasing video recording time to a total of 11 to 12 hours.[18,23,28–30]

OMOM

The OMOM system (Jianshan Science and Technology Group Co, Ltd, Chongqing, China) is the last commercially available VCE system. It measures 13 × 28 mm in size, has a 140° field of view, captures images at 2 frames per second using a complementary metal-oxide semiconductor, and has an 8-hour battery life. This system is accompanied by reading software with a "Similar Pictures Elimination Mode" intended to decrease the reading time required for a study. In a study of 200 patients undergoing OMOM VCE, using level 1 (low) "Similar Pictures Elimination Mode," there was similar sensitivity of the study compared with the conventional mode; however, there was a marked decrease in sensitivity when increasing to levels 2 or 3 (medium or high).[31,32]

Comparison of Video Capsule Endoscopy Systems

There are multiple studies comparing the diagnostic yield of different VCE systems. The primary limitation of all of these studies is the emergence of newer versions of each VCE system after publication. Therefore, no specific conclusions can be drawn favoring one VCE system over another, but rather each system will have its own attributes and limitations, which should be weighed by the individual provider when deciding which system is most ideal for each institution.

The original generation PillCam SB1 and Endocapsule systems were compared in a total of 51 patients undergoing tandem VCE studies for obscure gastrointestinal bleeding, which showed a comparable diagnostic yield between the 2 VCE systems.[22] In a study of 60 patients undergoing tandem VCE for obscure gastrointestinal bleeding with PillCam SB2 (Given Imaging) and the 4-camera CapsoCam SV-1 (CapsoVision), there was comparable identification of positive patients (84.8% PillCam SB2 vs 81.8% CapsoCam SV-1; $P = .791$), although CapsoCam SV-1 did detect significantly more lesions overall (108 vs 85; $P = .001$).[16]

Again using a tandem approach, the PillCam SB2 and MiroCam were compared in 2 studies of 105 and 83 patients for obscure gastrointestinal bleeding, which found reasonable concordance rates for positive findings among both capsule subtypes, but a significantly longer duration of video for MiroCam than PillCam SB2.[17,18] The MiroCam and Endocapsule systems have been compared in 50 patients undergoing VCE for a variety of indications, showing no significant differences in terms of completion rate of study to cecum and of diagnostic yield. Even with moderate concordance for diagnostic yield, both systems had several missed findings.[23]

Additional Video Capsule Endoscopy Hardware and Software Features

Standard VCE devices have traditionally recorded approximately 8 hours of video. More recently, newer generations of some VCE systems have increased recording times from 8 hours up to 12 to 15 hours, with a resulting increase in completion rate of VCE reaching the cecum by between 4% and 8%, although no significant change in diagnostic yield of the study.[33,34] The importance, however, of a complete VCE study cannot be overemphasized because it provides certainty of diagnosis to both the patient and the provider. Even with a complete VCE study, VCE may still miss 20% to 30% of lesions, and VCE may need to be repeated if the study is incomplete or reported as normal but with high clinical suspicion for ongoing small bowel abnormality.

Currently, there are commercially available, externally controlled VCE systems. The MiroCam Navi (IntroMedic) is able to be maneuvered using extracorporeal magnets to control VCE movement through the stomach and enable improved gastric visualization.[35] The goal of this type of system is to potentially serve as a substitute for endoscopic evaluation of the stomach.[36,37] These systems are not designed to be able to provide VCE control of movement through the small bowel.

Enhancements to software reading programs to improve diagnostic yield have also been proposed. Similar to chromoendoscopy that is used for lesion enhancement in the colon during colonoscopy, efforts have been made to develop forms of virtual chromoendoscopy to highlight lesions in the small bowel. These image processing algorithms include a flexible spectral imaging color enhancement and use a blue filter as part of the Rapid software with PillCam.[38–42] Some of these programs have shown promise, but further study of this type of image processing overall is needed before consideration for widespread adoption in conventional VCE reading.

READING A VIDEO CAPSULE ENDOSCOPY STUDY

First and most importantly, the VCE reader should know the indication and relevant clinical history to potentially guide interpretation. This is especially important in larger practices where capsules are read by a provider not directly involved in care of the particular patient or in situations where the VCE is sent out for reading. The initial phase for VCE reading is identification of anatomic landmarks, which should then be recorded in the VCE study report. These landmarks include first gastric image, first duodenal image, and first cecal image at a minimum. The presence of villi only in small bowel tissue may assist in distinction of transitions from gastric to small bowel images and then from small bowel to colonic images. Identification of the first ileocecal image may have high interobserver variability. Visualized features such as "Barkin Lines," also known as ileal lines, which are a grouping of parallel red lines that merge forming a rosette-type pattern at the ileocecal valve, may aid in the identification of the ileocecal valve and help standardize reading[43] (**Fig. 1**).

The second phase in VCE reading is determination of SBTT, which is calculated by subtracting the time of the first duodenal image from the first cecal image, previously marked as identified anatomic landmarks. Calculation of SBTT is done automatically in most VCE reading programs. Rapid SBTT of less than 2 hours may lead to missed lesions.[44] This, however, does not take into account newer VCE devices with variable frame rates and increased number of cameras with higher frame rates, which may be able to overcome the effects of rapid transit.

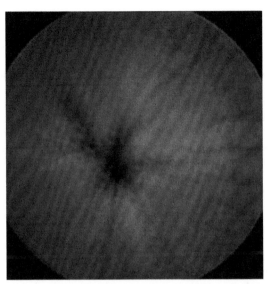

Fig. 1. Ileal lines are a grouping of parallel red lines that merge forming a rosette-type pattern at the ileocecal valve. (*Reprinted from* Carrion AF, Hindi M, Molina E, et al. Ileal lines: a marker of the ileocecal valve on wireless capsule endoscopy. Gastrointest Endosc 2014;79(5):871–2; with permission.)

If there are abnormal findings during VCE, the percent of SBTT will, if needed, guide the subsequent endoscopic approach for intervention. An anterograde approach for enteroscopy is used if the lesion is located within the first two-thirds of the SBTT, and a retrograde approach is preferred if more than two-thirds of the SBTT. It is important to provide a detailed description of VCE findings and include VCE images in the reports. When lesions are encountered, they should be classified using the Saurin classification system, where P2 indicates a definite lesion (angiodysplastic lesion, ulceration, or neoplasm) and P1 signifies a finding of unclear certainty (red spot or erosion).[45] Some VCE software programs may also feature VCE atlases, which serve as a consultative device for VCE readers trying to classify a challenging image.

The quality of small bowel preparation should be assessed in each third of the small bowel, which is based on the ability to visualize the entire small bowel lumen not obscured by bubbles or other debris. Quality of preparation may be quantified using a reader-assigned or computer-assigned cleanliness percentage scale.[46] More recently, quality of bowel preparation was examined using both a subjective score based on a modified Boston Bowel Preparation Scale and an objective assessment of percentage of mucosa obscured. There was lack of correlation between the subjective and objective scores, and assessment of bowel preparation using objective scoring based on percentage of obscured mucosa was favored as a marker of VCE study quality.[47]

The primary aim of VCE remains visualization of the small bowel; however, careful examination of gastric and colonic images to look for otherwise missed lesions is critical, especially in patients with obscure gastrointestinal bleeding. In patients with obscure gastrointestinal bleeding, VCE may detect up to 25% of upper gastrointestinal lesions in the esophagus and stomach that were not previously identified on upper endoscopy.[48–51]

Reader fatigue plays a role in the diagnostic yield of a VCE study. The impact of reader fatigue is similar to changes in adenoma detection rate, which may occur in late-in-the-day colonoscopies. Therefore, reading VCE studies throughout the day as opposed to the end of the day if possible may be preferred, and consideration against reading multiple VCE studies consecutively to minimize reader fatigue should be undertaken.

VCE studies can be read at a variety of frame rates and image modes with single or multiple images at once. Single-image reading at 10 frames per second is comparable to a 4-image view at a speed of 20 frames per second with similar diagnostic yield, and associated decreased reading time.[52,53] Reading rates over 15 to 20 frames per second are not routinely recommended as lesions may be missed.[54]

TROUBLESHOOTING IN VIDEO CAPSULE ENDOSCOPY

Counseling and a clear informed consent process with the patient and/or guardian is of utmost importance in VCE as in any other gastrointestinal procedure. The lack of sedation for this procedure does not change the necessity for informed consent, and a discussion of the technical procedural description, risks, benefits, and alternatives is mandatory. If a recording device is attached to the patient, discussion of removal time and activities such as bathing while the device is attached is required. Although perhaps lower than other more intervention-based gastroenterologic procedures oftentimes requiring sedation and its additional associated risks, the risks of VCE are by no means trivial.

RISKS OF VIDEO CAPSULE ENDOSCOPY

There are multiple potential risks of VCE. First, aspiration of the capsule itself or of the liquid used to facilitate swallowing of the capsule may occur. In the case of aspiration of the capsule itself, prompt referral for bronchoscopy and retrieval should be undertaken. Furthermore, the VCE may become lodged in a previously unknown Zenker diverticulum and remain as a retained foreign body.[55] Therefore, sore throat, dysphagia, odynophagia, dyspnea, or wheezing after VCE administration requires further evaluation.

Perhaps the most common risk of VCE is retention, defined as nonpassage of VCE into the cecum with 2 weeks of administration.[56] Retention rates are estimated to be 1% to 2% in patients with suspected small bowel bleeding, most commonly due to small bowel neoplasms, strictures due to usage of nonsteroidal anti-inflammatory drugs, radiation enteritis, prior surgical anastomoses, or inflammatory bowel disease (IBD).[57–62] Importantly, in patients with IBD, the risk of VCE retention may increase from 2% up to 13% in some series.[57,59,62,63]

Patients with increased potential for VCE retention should undergo further evaluation of luminal patency before VCE administration using computed tomography (CT) or magnetic resonance (MR) enterography. Unfortunately, a normal enterography does not completely rule out the potential for retention because lesions, such as nonsteroidal induced small bowel diaphragms and IBD-associated localized strictures, may be missed. A swallowed PillCam patency capsule (Given Imaging) should be used for further evaluation before VCE in administration in these high-risk patients. The patency capsule is composed of a dissolvable lactose body and a radiofrequency identification (RFID) tag. The patient can be scanned 30 hours after patency capsule administration to evaluate for the presence of the RFID tag, indicating possible increased risk for subsequent VCE retention.[64]

In the setting of a small bowel obstruction, there is a chance of the VCE causing perforation if the capsule impacts and eventually erodes at the obstruction site. There is also one report of a VCE impacting in the appendiceal orifice leading to an acute appendicitis.[65] The patient should be asymptomatic after VCE. If abdominal pain occurs after VCE administration, small bowel stenosis or obstruction should be suspected.

The risk of a retained capsule remains an ongoing concern. Consideration before VCE is warranted as to whether the patient would be able to tolerate an endoscopic procedure for both capsule retrieval if needed and also to intervene on any encountered lesions. In otherwise asymptomatic patients, an abdominal radiograph should be obtained if there is no evidence of capsule passage into the colon at the end of the video recording, associated with no witnessed capsule passage per rectum or ostomy by the patient within 14 days of capsule administration. In the case of patients found to have a retained capsule and who are symptomatic, prompt retrieval or removal should be undertaken, preferably from an endoscopic approach using enteroscopy, and potentially via surgery if an endoscopic approach is not feasible or successful. Capsule retention always indicates an anatomic cause of the nonpassage.

CONTRAINDICATIONS TO VIDEO CAPSULE ENDOSCOPY

There are multiple contraindications to VCE administration, both relative and absolute. A known and symptomatic luminal obstruction or ileus should be considered as the only absolute contraindication to VCE. Pregnancy is a relative contraindication due to the elevated risk to the fetus if capsule retrieval is required. Crohn's disease with known or highly suspected small bowel stricturing disease should be viewed as a relative contraindication. In this subgroup of patients, consideration of a patency capsule and/or further abdominal imaging including CT or MR enterography before VCE to evaluate for strictures should be strongly considered. Altered mental status in a patient causing inability to follow commands is a relative contraindication, as oral VCE administration may be high risk with nonswallowing of the VCE or its aspiration, and the potential yield of the study may be compromised if the patient unwittingly removes the recording device before completion of the study.

Advanced age should not be considered a contraindication to VCE. Similarly, low VCE adverse event rates of approximately 1% due to capsule retention in those less than and more than 80 years of age has been found.[66] Presence of an implantable cardiac device is not a contraindication to VCE, as VCE has been shown to be safe in these patients, although small adjustments to device settings may be needed before VCE.[67] However, the use of a magnetic controlled VCE device would remain contraindicated in this cohort because the magnet may interfere with the cardiac device.

TROUBLESHOOTING TIPS

- Approach the reading of VCE as you would with any other endoscopic procedure—alert, awake, and with knowledge of the patient.
- Remember the motto: Cleaner is better, to emphasize the importance of good bowel preparation.
- Administer prokinetic agents in some patients to improve gastric-emptying time and increase small bowel visualization time. Concomitant or prior use of simethicone may decrease bubbles and improve small bowel visualization.
- Encourage patients to be as active as possible, which improves capsule movement through the small bowel.
- Evaluate the patient for the presence of contraindications to VCE.

- In patients with suspected small bowel bleeding, time the capsule administration within 2 weeks of the bleeding event to increase diagnostic yield, and ideally the earlier after an acute event, the better.
- Some capsules may have a small screen to enable real-time viewing in select situations (such as a patient with concern for ongoing bleeding pending intervention) and may also help ensure a capsule has passed into the small bowel in patients in whom a prokinetic agent may be administered if the capsule remains in the stomach.

REFERENCES

1. Rokkas T, Papaxoinis K, Triantafyllou K, et al. Does purgative preparation influence the diagnostic yield of small bowel video capsule endoscopy?: a meta-analysis. Am J Gastroenterol 2009;104(1):219–27.
2. Park SC, Keum B, Seo YS, et al. Effect of bowel preparation with polyethylene glycol on quality of capsule endoscopy. Dig Dis Sci 2011;56(6):1769–75.
3. Rayner-Hartley E, Alsahafi M, Cramer P, et al. Low volume polyethylene glycol with ascorbic acid, sodium picosulfate-magnesium citrate, and clear liquid diet alone prior to small bowel capsule endoscopy. World J Gastrointest Endosc 2016;8(11):433–8.
4. Boal Carvalho P, Rosa B, Moreira MJ, et al. New evidence on the impact of antithrombotics in patients submitted to small bowel capsule endoscopy for the evaluation of obscure gastrointestinal bleeding. Gastroenterol Res Pract 2014;2014: 709217.
5. Van Weyenberg SJ, Van Turenhout ST, Jacobs MA, et al. Video capsule endoscopy for previous overt obscure gastrointestinal bleeding in patients using antithrombotic drugs. Dig Endosc 2012;24(4):247–54.
6. Rondonotti E, Herrerias JM, Pennazio M, et al. Complications, limitations, and failures of capsule endoscopy: a review of 733 cases. Gastrointest Endosc 2005; 62(5):712–6.
7. Westerhof J, Weersma RK, Koornstra JJ. Risk factors for incomplete small-bowel capsule endoscopy. Gastrointest Endosc 2009;69(1):74–80.
8. Stanich PP, Kleinman B, Porter KM, et al. Video capsule endoscopy after bariatric and gastric surgery: oral ingestion is associated with satisfactory completion rate. J Clin Gastroenterol 2015;49(1):31–3.
9. Shibuya T, Mori H, Takeda T, et al. The relationship between physical activity level and completion rate of small bowel examination in patients undergoing capsule endoscopy. Intern Med 2012;51(9):997–1001.
10. Bass LM, Misiewicz L. Use of a real-time viewer for endoscopic deployment of capsule endoscope in the pediatric population. J Pediatr Gastroenterol Nutr 2012;55(5):552–5.
11. Gibbs WB, Bloomfeld RS. Endoscopic deployment of video capsule endoscopy: does it guarantee a complete examination of the small bowel? Gastrointest Endosc 2012;76(4):905–9.
12. Gan HY, Weng YJ, Qiao WG, et al. Sedation with propofol has no effect on capsule endoscopy completion rates: a prospective single-center study. Medicine (Baltimore) 2015;94(27):e1140.
13. Westerhof J, Weersma RK, Hoedemaker RA, et al. Completion rate of small bowel capsule endoscopy is higher after erythromycin compared to domperidone. BMC Gastroenterol 2014;14:162.

14. Koulaouzidis A, Dimitriadis S, Douglas S, et al. The use of domperidone increases the completion rate of small bowel capsule endoscopy: does this come at the expense of diagnostic yield? J Clin Gastroenterol 2015;49(5):395–400.

15. Fernandez-Urien I, Carretero C, Borobio E, et al. Capsule endoscopy capture rate: has 4 frames-per-second any impact over 2 frames-per-second? World J Gastroenterol 2014;20(39):14472–8.

16. Pioche M, Vanbiervliet G, Jacob P, et al, French Society of Digestive Endoscopy (SFED). Prospective randomized comparison between axial- and lateral-viewing capsule endoscopy systems in patients with obscure digestive bleeding. Endoscopy 2014;46(6):479–84.

17. Choi EH, Mergener K, Semrad C, et al. A multicenter, prospective, randomized comparison of a novel signal transmission capsule endoscope to an existing capsule endoscope. Gastrointest Endosc 2013;78(2):325–32.

18. Pioche M, Gaudin JL, Filoche B, et al, French Society of Digestive Endoscopy. Prospective, randomized comparison of two small-bowel capsule endoscopy systems in patients with obscure GI bleeding. Gastrointest Endosc 2011;73(6):1181–8.

19. PillCam SB. Given imaging. 2016. Available at: http://www.givenimaging.com/en-us/Innovative-Solutions/Capsule-Endoscopy/Pillcam-SB/Pages/default.aspx. Accessed May 15, 2016.

20. Saurin JC, Ben Soussan E, Gaudric M, et al. Can we shorten the small-bowel capsule reading time? Validation of the "Quick-View" image detection system [abstract]. Gastrointest Endosc 2009;69:AB189.

21. Tal AO, Filmann N, Makhlin K, et al. The capsule endoscopy "suspected blood indicator" (SBI) for detection of active small bowel bleeding: no active bleeding in case of negative SBI. Scand J Gastroenterol 2014;49(9):1131–5.

22. Cave DR, Fleischer DE, Leighton JA, et al. A multicenter randomized comparison of the Endocapsule and the Pillcam SB. Gastrointest Endosc 2008;68(3):487–94.

23. Dolak W, Kulnigg-Dabsch S, Evstatiev R, et al. A randomized head-to-head study of small-bowel imaging comparing MiroCam and EndoCapsule. Endoscopy 2012;44(11):1012–20.

24. ENDOCAPSULE 10 System - Olympus America – Medical. 2016. Available at: http://medical.olympusamerica.com/products/endocapsule-10-system. Accessed May 15, 2016.

25. Subramanian V, Mannath J, Telakis E, et al. Efficacy of new playback functions at reducing small-bowel wireless capsule endoscopy reading times. Dig Dis Sci 2012;57(6):1624–8.

26. Friedrich K, Gehrke S, Stremmel W, et al. First clinical trial of a newly developed capsule endoscope with panoramic side view for small bowel: a pilot study. J Gastroenterol Hepatol 2013;28(9):1496–501.

27. CapsoVision – CapsoCam. 2016. Available at: http://www.capsovision.com/index.php/capsocam.html. Accessed May 15, 2016.

28. Bang S, Park JY, Jeong S, et al. First clinical trial of the "MiRo" capsule endoscope by using a novel transmission technology: electric-field propagation. Gastrointest Endosc 2009;69(2):253–9.

29. Mussetto A, Fuccio L, Dari S, et al. MiroCam capsule for obscure gastrointestinal bleeding: a prospective, single centre experience. Dig Liver Dis 2013;45(2):124–8.

30. IntroMedic. 2016. Available at: http://www.intromedic.com/eng/sub_products_2.html. Accessed May 15, 2016.

31. OMOM capsule endoscopy system manufacturer from Chongqing China. 2016. Available at: http://jinshangroup.gmc.globalmarket.com/products/details/omom-capsule-endoscopy-system-4543846.html. Accessed May 15, 2016.

32. Xu Y, Zhang W, Ye S, et al. The evaluation of the OMOM capsule endoscopy with similar pictures elimination mode. Clin Res Hepatol Gastroenterol 2014;38(6):757–62.

33. Ou G, Shahidi N, Galorport C, et al. Effect of longer battery life on small bowel capsule endoscopy. World J Gastroenterol 2015;21(9):2677–82.

34. Rahman M, Akerman S, DeVito B, et al. Comparison of the diagnostic yield and outcomes between standard 8 h capsule endoscopy and the new 12 h capsule endoscopy for investigating small bowel pathology. World J Gastroenterol 2015; 21(18):5542–7.

35. Rahman I, Kay M, Bryant T, et al. Optimizing the performance of magnetic-assisted capsule endoscopy of the upper GI tract using multiplanar CT modeling. Eur J Gastroenterol Hepatol 2015;27(4):460–6.

36. Rey JF, Ogata H, Hosoe N, et al. Blinded nonrandomized comparative study of gastric examination with a magnetically guided capsule endoscope and standard videoendoscope. Gastrointest Endosc 2012;75(2):373–81.

37. Keller J, Fibbe C, Volke F, et al. Inspection of the human stomach using remote-controlled capsule endoscopy: a feasibility study in healthy volunteers (with videos). Gastrointest Endosc 2011;73(1):22–8.

38. Dias de Castro F, Magalhães J, Boal Carvalho P, et al. Improving diagnostic yield in obscure gastrointestinal bleeding–how virtual chromoendoscopy may be the answer. Eur J Gastroenterol Hepatol 2015;27(6):735–40.

39. Kobayashi Y, Watabe H, Yamada A, et al. Efficacy of flexible spectral imaging color enhancement on the detection of small intestinal diseases by capsule endoscopy. J Dig Dis 2012;13(12):614–20.

40. Krystallis C, Koulaouzidis A, Douglas S, et al. Chromoendoscopy in small bowel capsule endoscopy: blue mode or Fuji Intelligent Colour Enhancement? Dig Liver Dis 2011;43(12):953–7.

41. Boal Carvalho P, Magalhães J, Dias de Castro F, et al. Virtual chromoendoscopy improves the diagnostic yield of small bowel capsule endoscopy in obscure gastrointestinal bleeding. Dig Liver Dis 2016;48(2):172–5.

42. Imagawa H, Oka S, Tanaka S, et al. Improved detectability of small-bowel lesions via capsule endoscopy with computed virtual chromoendoscopy: a pilot study. Scand J Gastroenterol 2011;46(9):1133–7.

43. Carrion AF, Hindi M, Molina E, et al. Ileal lines: a marker of the ileocecal valve on wireless capsule endoscopy. Gastrointest Endosc 2014;79(5):871–2.

44. Buscaglia JM, Kapoor S, Clarke JO, et al. Enhanced diagnostic yield with prolonged small bowel transit time during capsule endoscopy. Int J Med Sci 2008; 5(6):303–8.

45. Saurin JC, Delvaux M, Gaudin JL, et al. Diagnostic value of endoscopic capsule in patients with obscure digestive bleeding: blinded comparison with video push-enteroscopy. Endoscopy 2003;35(7):576–84.

46. Hong-Bin C, Yue H, Su-Yu C, et al. Evaluation of visualized area percentage assessment of cleansing score and computed assessment of cleansing score for capsule endoscopy. Saudi J Gastroenterol 2013;19(4):160–4.

47. Barkin JA, Chen CH, Barkin JS, et al. Coast to coast quality indicators for video capsule endoscopy. Presented at American College of Gastroenterology Annual Scientific Meeting, October 14–19, 2016, Las Vegas, Nevada. Poster 1396.

48. Lepileur L, Dray X, Antonietti M, et al. Factors associated with diagnosis of obscure gastrointestinal bleeding by video capsule enteroscopy. Clin Gastroenterol Hepatol 2012;10(12):1376–80.

49. Gerson LB. Outcomes associated with deep enteroscopy. Gastrointest Endosc Clin N Am 2009;19(3):481–96.

50. Gerson LB, Fidler JL, Cave DR, et al. ACG Clinical Guideline: diagnosis and management of small bowel bleeding. Am J Gastroenterol 2015;110(9):1265–87.
51. Tacheci I, Devière J, Kopacova M, et al. The importance of upper gastrointestinal lesions detected with capsule endoscopy in patients with obscure digestive bleeding. Acta Gastroenterol Belg 2011;74(3):395–9.
52. Günther U, Daum S, Zeitz M, et al. Capsule endoscopy: comparison of two different reading modes. Int J Colorectal Dis 2012;27(4):521–5.
53. Kyriakos N, Karagiannis S, Galanis P, et al. Evaluation of four time-saving methods of reading capsule endoscopy videos. Eur J Gastroenterol Hepatol 2012;24(11):1276–80.
54. Zheng Y, Hawkins L, Wolff J, et al. Detection of lesions during capsule endoscopy: physician performance is disappointing. Am J Gastroenterol 2012;107(4):554–60.
55. Kropf JA, Jeanmonod R, Yen DM. An unusual presentation of a chronic ingested foreign body in an adult. J Emerg Med 2013;44(1):82–4.
56. Cave D, Legnani P, de Franchis R, et al. ICCE consensus for capsule retention. Endoscopy 2005;37(10):1065–7.
57. Liao Z, Gao R, Xu C, et al. Indications and detection, completion, and retention rates of small-bowel capsule endoscopy: a systematic review. Gastrointest Endosc 2010;71(2):280–6.
58. Li F, Gurudu SR, De Petris G, et al. Retention of the capsule endoscope: a single-center experience of 1000 capsule endoscopy procedures. Gastrointest Endosc 2008;68(1):174–80.
59. Cheifetz AS, Kornbluth AA, Legnani P, et al. The risk of retention of the capsule endoscope in patients with known or suspected Crohn's disease. Am J Gastroenterol 2006;101(10):2218–22.
60. Rondonotti E, Pennazio M, Toth E, et al, European Capsule Endoscopy Group, Italian Club for Capsule Endoscopy (CICE), Iberian Group for Capsule Endoscopy. Small-bowel neoplasms in patients undergoing video capsule endoscopy: a multicenter European study. Endoscopy 2008;40(6):488–95.
61. Höög CM, Bark LÅ, Arkani J, et al. Capsule retentions and incomplete capsule endoscopy examinations: an analysis of 2300 examinations. Gastroenterol Res Pract 2012;2012:518718.
62. Cheon JH, Kim YS, Lee IS, et al, Korean Gut Image Study Group. Can we predict spontaneous capsule passage after retention? A nationwide study to evaluate the incidence and clinical outcomes of capsule retention. Endoscopy 2007;39(12):1046–52.
63. Pennazio M, Spada C, Eliakim R, et al. Small-bowel capsule endoscopy and device-assisted enteroscopy for diagnosis and treatment of small-bowel disorders: European Society of Gastrointestinal Endoscopy (ESGE) Clinical Guideline. Endoscopy 2015;47(4):352–76.
64. Caunedo-Alvarez A, Romero-Vazquez J, Herrerias-Gutierrez JM. Patency and agile capsules. World J Gastroenterol 2008;14(34):5269–73.
65. Matta A, Koppala J, Reddymasu SC, et al. Acute appendicitis: a potential complication of video capsule endoscopy. BMJ Case Rep 2014;2014. http://dx.doi.org/10.1136/bcr-2014-204240.
66. Gómez V, Cheesman AR, Heckman MG, et al. Safety of capsule endoscopy in the octogenarian as compared with younger patients. Gastrointest Endosc 2013;78(5):744–9.
67. Stanich PP, Kleinman B, Betkerur K, et al. Video capsule endoscopy is successful and effective in outpatients with implantable cardiac devices. Dig Endosc 2014;26(6):726–30.

Small Bowel Capsule Endoscopy

Normal Findings and Normal Variants of the Small Bowel

Marco Pennazio, MD[a],*, Emanuele Rondonotti, MD, PhD[b],
Anastasios Koulaouzidis, MD, FACG, FRCPE[c]

KEYWORDS

- Capsule endoscopy • Normal small bowel • Anatomic landmarks
- Variants of normal • Artifacts • Lymphangiectasias • Angioectasia • Bulges

KEY POINTS

- Recognizing typical anatomic landmarks as well as distinguishing normal small bowel anatomy from abnormal findings on small bowel capsule endoscopy (SBCE) may be challenging, especially for novice readers.
- The reader of capsule images may often encounter unusual views of the normal anatomy and various artifacts that need to be recognized and distinguished from pathologic findings; small, innocent findings should not be overinterpreted.
- Experience gained through standard endoscopy is invaluable to the interpretation of SBCE examinations; however, formalized training and credentialing in reading competency are essential.

INTRODUCTION

Small bowel capsule endoscopy (SBCE) is fundamentally different from conventional flexible endoscopy, albeit still digestive endoscopy. Differentiating normal from abnormal in SBCE is not always as easy as it sounds; often it is hampered by the lack of control over the capsule movement and/or the direction of view. Furthermore, the inability to carry out typical maneuvers of conventional endoscopy, such as

Disclosure Statements: The authors do not declare any commercial or financial conflict of interest and any funding sources related to this work.
Author Contributions: M. Pennazio substantially contributed to the article conception and drafted the paper; A. Koulaouzids and E. Rondonotti supervised the work and revised it critically for important intellectual content. All the authors approved the final version.
[a] Division of Gastroenterology U, San Giovanni AS University-Teaching Hospital, Via Cavour 31, Torino 10123, Italy; [b] Gastroenterology Unit, Valduce Hospital, Via Dante 11, Como 22100, Italy; [c] The Royal Infirmary of Edinburgh, Edinburgh EH16 4SA, UK
* Corresponding author.
E-mail address: pennazio.marco@gmail.com

Gastrointest Endoscopy Clin N Am 27 (2017) 29–50
http://dx.doi.org/10.1016/j.giec.2016.08.003
1052-5157/17/© 2016 Elsevier Inc. All rights reserved.

giendo.theclinics.com

suctioning, flushing, or simply biopsying in case of uncertainty, represents one of the major limitations of current SBCE. Therefore, diagnosis or even a presumptive one is often based solely on the images captured by the video capsule. Normal variants and nonpathologic findings must also be clearly recognized. Hence, when interpreting SBCE, some special features of this diagnostic modality should be taken into account; that is, the image is more magnified than the image obtained with conventional endoscopy, and therefore, small innocent findings should not be overrated. The SBCE readers should also be familiar with technical details of different available capsules, which differ for number and location of cameras (ie, the recently introduced panoramic lateral-viewing capsule provide a tape view instead of the tubular view of frontal viewing capsules), field of view, depth of view, battery duration, and image capture rate. Experience gained through standard digestive endoscopy is certainly invaluable to the interpretation of SBCE videos; nevertheless, formalized training and credentialing in SBCE reading competency are also essential.[1]

This article deals with the normal anatomy of the small bowel as realized by SBCE as well as some artifacts and normal variants that may be found during a capsule examination; the reader should become familiar with the latter in order to be able to distinguish them from pathologic findings.

ESOPHAGEAL AND GASTRIC PASSAGE

Although SBCE is an examination primarily devoted to the study of the small bowel, useful information can sometimes be extracted from the esophageal and gastric portion of the study. In addition, although SBCE has some inherent limitations in the study of the stomach and the esophagus, the SBCE readers have to inspect these organs because obvious clinically relevant findings, missed by previous gastroscopies, are discovered in the upper gastrointestinal (GI) tract in up to 15% of SBCE examinations.

The capsule records images of the mouth and oropharynx, but they are limited and not adequate for making a formal diagnosis. The upper esophageal sphincter is rarely identified, whereas the rest of the esophagus only occasionally can be reliably evaluated because of the exceptionally swift passage of the capsule. The first images of the esophagus show a dark hollow tube (**Fig. 1**). The squamous epithelium lining appears pale white; the vessels beneath the epithelium are seen as tiny pale red curly lines (**Fig. 2**). In the normal esophagus, the Z-line is coincident with the gastroesophageal junction, defined as the upper end of the gastric folds. The Z-line is shortly visualized during the examination in most patients (**Fig. 3**). It can display different shapes: round, starlike, flamelike, blurry, and/or distorted. Complete visualization of the Z-line is often challenging because the individual frames obtained might include only a portion of it. Z-line visualization can be accurately achieved in most cases if the patient swallows the capsule while lying in the right supine position[2] or when dual cameras with higher image capture rate (ie, PillCam Colon Capsule 2 [Pill Cam, Medtronic, Minneapolis, MN]) are used.

Pathologic findings are occasionally seen, most commonly at the Z-line: when they are well demarcated such as Barrett's esophagus or esophagitis, they should be described but need clarification by additional investigations such as esophagogastroduodenoscopy.

The first gastric image is usually dark, given the wide space present in the gastric cavity. Passage into the stomach is featured by several rapid changes in the capsule direction. Typical passage times of the capsule in the stomach range from a few minutes to 1 hour. Similarly to the esophagus, the gastric mucosa is incompletely visualized at SBCE, and this examination cannot substitute for examining the upper GI tract by esophagogastroduodenoscopy, when clinically indicated. Attention to the

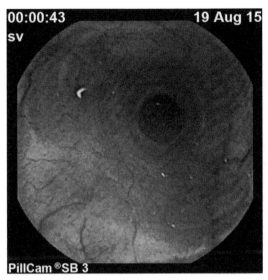

Fig. 1. Broad vision of the normal esophagus.

surface structure of the gastric mucosa, that generally appears smooth and some-times exhibits a mosaic pattern (**Fig. 4**), can provide important clues, especially for its differentiation from the mucosa of the duodenal bulb.

SUBDIVISION OF THE SMALL BOWEL

The small bowel is a tubular organ up to 5 m long, which starts at the pylorus and ends at the ileocecal valve. It is subdivided into the duodenum, the jejunum, and the ileum. Although there are some differences in structure between jejunum and ileum, a precise

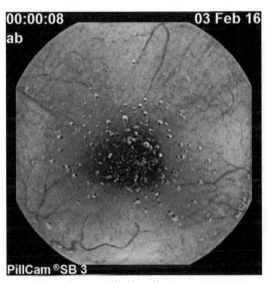

Fig. 2. Detail of the normal esophagus with the pale silvery appearance and vascular pattern.

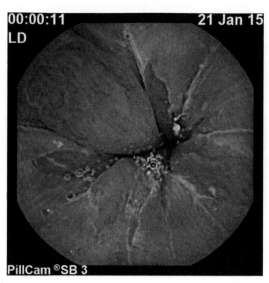

Fig. 3. Normal Z-line.

transition cannot be defined; however, the duodenum and terminal ileum can be iden-tified easily. The localization software of capsule endoscopy is occasionally helpful in distinguishing the distal duodenum from the jejunum and the terminal ileum from the mid ileum. Therefore, in SBCE interpretation, the subdivision of the small bowel is based mostly on pragmatic considerations. The time that elapses between the pylorus and the first cecal image is divided into 3 equal parts. The small bowel segments in SBCE may thus be enumerated in this way: duodenum, proximal third of the small bowel, middle third of the small bowel, distal third of the small bowel, and terminal

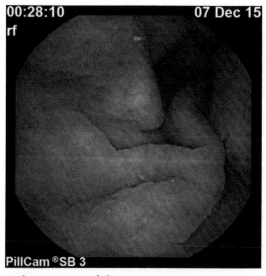

Fig. 4. Normal mucosal appearance of the gastric antrum.

ileum. The position of the capsule or any identified abnormality can also be reported by indicating the time that has elapsed between the passage of the imaging device through the pylorus and its current position, thereby estimating its position in the "proximal" or "distal" portion of the small bowel.[3,4]

PYLORUS AND DUODENAL BULB

The typical aspect of the pylorus is easily recognized at capsule endoscopy (**Fig. 5**) and, while the capsule is still in the stomach, it is occasionally possible to get a trans-pyloric view into the duodenal bulb (**Fig. 6**). If the capsule is pointing in a favorable direction, the distal aspect of the pylorus may be visible from within the bulb as a circular ridge (**Fig. 7**). In this situation, the mucosa of the pylorus appears flat, whereas the surrounding mucosa of the duodenum is covered by villi (**Fig. 8**). Therefore, the somewhat protuberant appearance of the pylorus in this view should not be mistaken for a polyp or mass lesion (**Fig. 9**). A back-and-forth movement across the pylorus may also occasionally be observed with retrograde passage of the capsule from the duodenal bulb into the stomach and then again into the bulb. Views of the duodenal bulb are usually brief. Unlike the gastric mucosa, the duodenal bulb typically reveals superficial breaks and fissures that correspond histologically to the presence of crypts (see **Fig. 8**). At this level, the presence of fluid, bile, and food particles may obscure luminal views and hamper the correct interpretation of the device location.

Single or multiple small nodules, representing Brunner glands, are a typical feature of the duodenum, but they can also be found in the descending duodenum. Foci of heterotopic gastric mucosa may also present as discrete nodules or multiple sessile polyps in the duodenum (**Fig. 10**). Both conditions are typically asymptomatic and discovered incidentally; their differentiation requires histologic evaluation by biopsy specimens.

Folds are first seen past the apex of the bulb, and circular folds first appear in the descending duodenum. Bile is usually visible in the bowel lumen at this level.

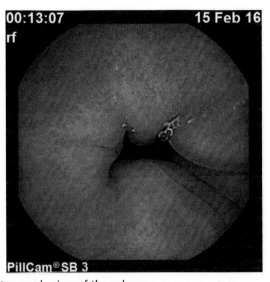

Fig. 5. Normal anterograde view of the pylorus.

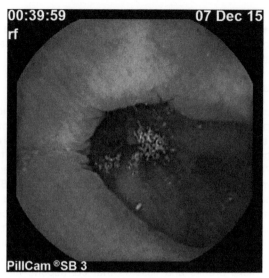

Fig. 6. View through the pylorus into the duodenal bulb.

PAPILLA OF VATER AND MINOR PAPILLA

The major papilla, also termed papilla of Vater, is difficult to identify in the nondistended duodenum; it is sometimes concealed by luminal content such as bile or may be missed due to the quick duodenal passage of the capsule. It is imaged in approximately 10% of patients during SBCE[5] with frontal viewing capsules and up to 70% in SBCE with lateral panoramic view (CapsoCam, CapsoVision, Cupertino, California).[6] If identified, the major papilla appears as a small nodule with a central pinpoint or slitlike opening that is sometimes marked by the drainage of bile (**Figs.**

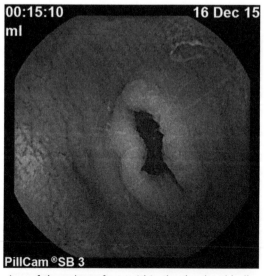

Fig. 7. Retrograde view of the pylorus from within the duodenal bulb.

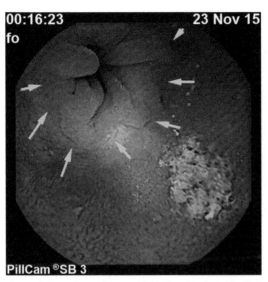

Fig. 8. Retrograde view of the pylorus from within the duodenal bulb (*arrows* indicate the transition point between the mucosa of the pylorus and that of the duodenal bulb).

11 and **12**). The minor papilla, which is located just proximal to the papilla of Vater, is even more rarely seen. Time after ingestion to reach the papilla of Vater is quite variable, as is the time interval between passage through the pylorus to the papilla. Usually this takes only seconds to a few minutes, but rarely, prolonged stay of the capsule in the duodenum or retroperistalsis may cause visualization of the papilla up to I or 2 hours after it passes the pylorus.

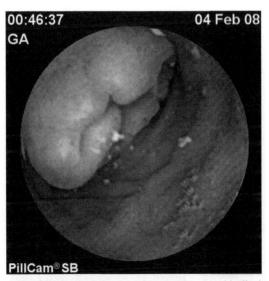

Fig. 9. Retrograde view of the pylorus from within the duodenal bulb showing a particular protuberant appearance of the pylorus.

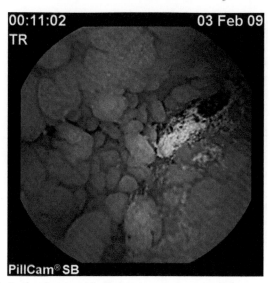

Fig. 10. Nodularity in the duodenal bulb due to gastric metaplasia.

NORMAL VIDEO CAPSULE ENDOSCOPY OF THE SMALL BOWEL

There are various characteristics of the "normal" small bowel shown by SBCE: the mucosa is usually yellow-orange–colored; normal findings are also the circular folds (valvulae conniventes), the villi, small vessels and occasionally larger veins, bile, air bubbles and debris in secretions, and Peyer patches in the terminal ileum.

The valvulae conniventes are more prominent and closely spaced in the duodenum and jejunum (**Fig. 13**A), are less well developed, and more widely separated in the ileum (**Fig. 13**B), although there is not a clear-cut transition zone; they are absent

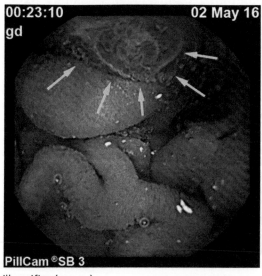

Fig. 11. Major papilla orifice (*arrows*).

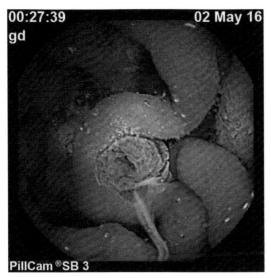

Fig. 12. Major papilla.

from the terminal ileum. White lines are a normal feature of small intestinal mucosa: they are sometimes observed at the edges of the folds and probably are in relation to their various states of contraction because the intestinal lumen is not distended during the examination (**Fig. 14**). The high resolution of SBCE provides a detailed view of the bowel mucosa, including the mucosal villi: in the fluid-filled small bowel, these fingerlike structures can be very clearly seen and evaluated when viewed at a tangential angle (see **Figs. 12** and **13**A). Villi are tallest in the jejunum and progressively shorter in the ileum. Nevertheless, the jejunum and ileum cannot be reliably distinguished in SBCE just by the appearance of their villi. Blood vessels are most clearly

A   **B**

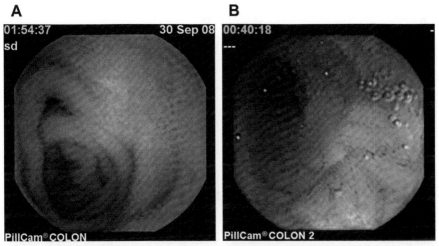

Fig. 13. Circumferential mucosal folds are more dense and prominent in the jejunum (A) than in the ileum (B).

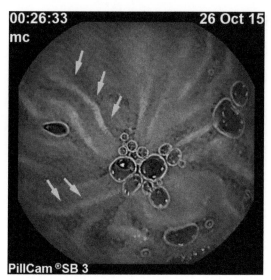

Fig. 14. White lines (indicated by *arrows*) observed at the edges of normal folds in a non-distended small bowel.

visualized when viewed directly from above. The vascular pattern in the ileum is more distinct than in the other segments (**Fig. 15**).

The small bowel shows brisk peristaltic activity, recognized by the contraction and migration of the valvulae conniventes and small, superimposed folds. The contractions show varying temporal patterns, with smaller bidirectional movements and intermittent forceful, propulsive contractions. For these reasons, it is not unusual for a capsule to move forward and backward, caught in a mixing cycle only then to ride a peristaltic wave distally. This phenomenon also explains the variability of small bowel passage times even when examinations are repeated in the same patient. For those who interpret SBCE examinations, it is important to know that this to-and-fro motion may limit the

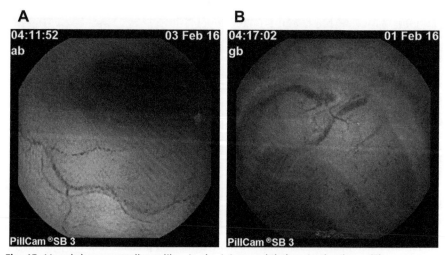

Fig. 15. Vessels have a smaller caliber in the jejunum (*A*) than in the ileum (*B*).

ability of the capsule to accurately count the number of lesions seen whether vascular lesions or mucosal breaks, and may also mimic the presence of multiple lesions.

Several artifacts can be discovered during the video analysis. An occasional situation that should not be confused with a pathologic finding is when, especially during rapid transit of the device, the intestinal lumen appears collapsed, precluding the normal small bowel visualization (**Fig. 16**); moreover, when the small intestine mucosa is displayed through an air bubble, some translucent lines may appear, representing the air/water interface on the edge of a large bubble (**Fig. 17**); this light reflection can give the false impression of absent villi. The analysis of the moving video images is useful to identify and clarify this phenomenon. A reflection of light close to the air/water interface may also provide a clue. Sometimes, the front light sources of the capsule may be reflected in these air bubbles (**Fig. 18**). The clarity of the capsule images depends on the distance of the imaging device from the bowel wall and the presence or absence of fluid or debris inside the lumen of the small intestine. The intraluminal fluid is more concentrated in the ileum and, for its content of bile, the vision is darker in the distal ileum compared with the proximal small intestine. Dark bile is thus a situation that can be difficult for the beginning reader, who can mistake bile for dark blood (**Fig. 19**). This error is avoided by examining the mucosa beyond the stained area to look for "coffee grounds" or bloody material. Their absence indicates likely bile proximally.

TERMINAL ILEUM AND ILEOCECAL VALVE

A characteristic feature of the terminal ileum is the presence of multiple small (2–3 mm) lymphoid follicles (**Fig. 20**). They are more prominent during childhood and adolescence but may be seen at all ages and should not be mistaken for polyps. Reflux of colonic content can frequently be observed during capsule examinations and may sometimes preclude adequate visualization of the distal aspect of the terminal ileum. At the ileocecal valve, sometimes longitudinal, stretched vessels are seen (**Fig. 21**), and villi may become scattered at this transition zone between the small and large

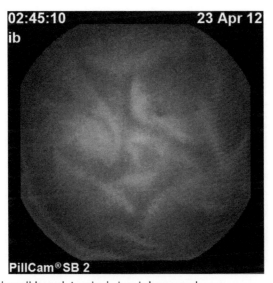

Fig. 16. Collapsed small bowel. Luminal view is hampered.

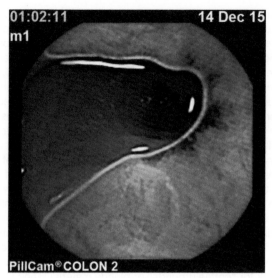

Fig. 17. Artifact lines created at the air/water interface of a large air bubble.

intestines (**Fig. 22**). The capsule may move back and forth in the terminal ileum for some time. Passage of the capsule through the valve itself is usually very abrupt, yielding only an initial image of the colon.

DIFFERENTIATING INCIDENTAL FINDINGS FROM PATHOLOGIC ONES

There may be several incidental findings detected at SBCE; some of them are frequent and do not represent abnormality of clinical significance. In some special cases, given

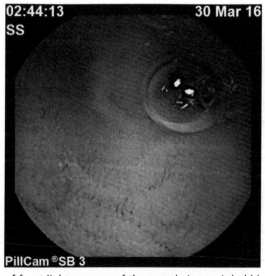

Fig. 18. Reflection of front lights sources of the capsule in an air bubble.

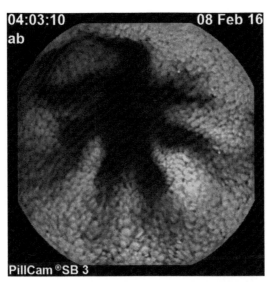

Fig. 19. Dark fluid in the distal small bowel can be mistaken for dark blood.

the significant clinical consequences of an erroneous diagnosis, good expertise is required to differentiate what is a normal finding from a pathologic lesion.

LYMPHANGIECTASIAS

Endoscopically, the villi of the small bowel in intestinal lymphangiectasia typically appear white and may be swollen. The whitish discoloration of the villi is caused by chylomicrons, which accumulate in and obstruct the dilated lymphatic capillaries. Lymphangiectasias may be single, patchy, or diffuse. When involving the small

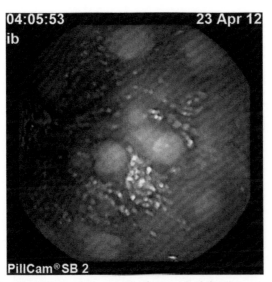

Fig. 20. Nodular lymphoid hyperplasia seen in the terminal ileum.

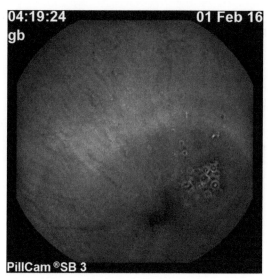

Fig. 21. Longitudinal stretched vessels at the ileocecal valve.

lacteals of individual villi, tiny punctate white spots may be seen on the mucosal surface (**Fig. 23**A); they are more common in the proximal small bowel. Clustering of such lymphangiectasias may present as bright white nodular protrusions (**Fig. 23**B). Cystic dilations of larger lymph vessels in the mucosa and submucosa of the bowel wall are referred to as chylous (lymphangiectatic) cysts or cholesterol cysts. They are yellow-white–colored, irregularly shaped, flat or raised into the bowel lumen with (pseudo) polypoid appearance, and with the submucosal vessels often clearly visible (**Fig. 23**C). All these forms are usually found incidentally and have not been shown

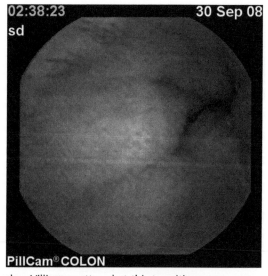

Fig. 22. Ileocecal valve. Villi are scattered at this transition zone.

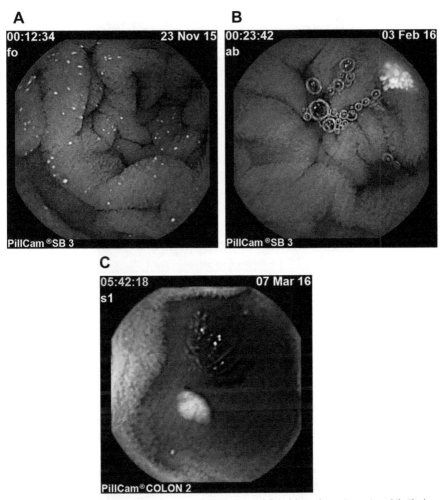

Fig. 23. (*A*) Punctate lymphangiectasias. (*B*) Cluster of focal lymphangiectasias. (*C*) Chylous cyst.

to have pathologic significance. A more diffuse whitish appearance of the small bowel mucosa can occasionally be observed during SBCE (**Fig. 24**), sometimes in otherwise asymptomatic individuals; it is perhaps dependent on food intake and appears to have no pathologic significance. Diffuse lymphangiectasia, as can be observed in Waldmann disease,[7] causes protein loss, and the mucosa appears "snow covered" or "dusted with powdered sugar" at SBCE (**Fig. 25**). Biopsy confirmation is advised.

PHLEBECTASIAS

Small venous ectasias, also called phlebectasias, are frequently seen during SBCE of the normal small bowel. Phlebectasias of different sizes can be found isolated (**Fig. 26**) or multiple, appearing as bluish vascular dilatations that are not raised like a small bowel varix or those protruding and with irregular surface of the blue rubber bleb nevus syndrome.[8] When they are small, they probably represent incidental findings

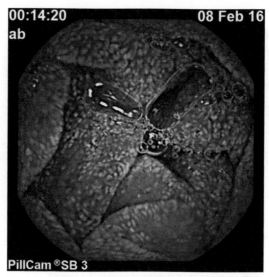

Fig. 24. Functional lymphangiectasia with whitish appearance of the mucosa in the jejunum.

without clinical significance. Conversely, large venous ectasias with an eroded surface should be considered a potential bleeding source.

BULGES

One of the most challenging tasks in reviewing capsule images is the evaluation of single-image abnormalities and proper identification of submucosal processes. Unlike traditional endoscopy, a single-image abnormality cannot be viewed from different

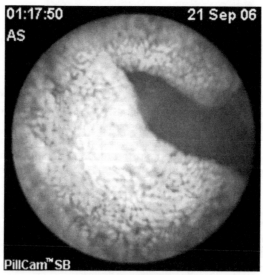

Fig. 25. Diffuse lymphangiectasias (Waldmann disease).

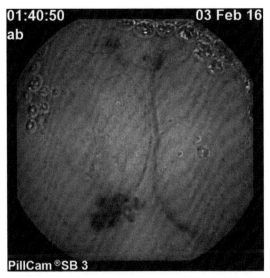

Fig. 26. Small phlebectasia.

angles but rather must be identified by a single, half-second image. A particularly complex situation is the distinction between a small bowel submucosal tumor and an innocent bulge, especially if luminal views are suboptimal and only a few capsule images show the area in question. A bulge is defined as a round and smooth, large base protrusion in the lumen having an ill-defined edge on the surrounding mucosa; it can be a prominent normal fold, a loop of bowel overlying the loop being inspected (ie, an extrinsic compression), or the luminal expression of intestinal loop angulation and stiffness. Sometimes, it can be virtually indistinguishable from a small submucosal tumor. Overlying loops or adjacent organs can be suspected when the protrusion moves with peristalsis, indicating its softness and extrinsic location (**Fig. 27**A). In this situation, the

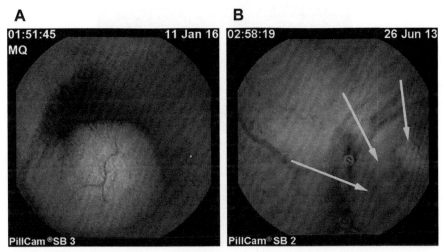

Fig. 27. (A) Innocent small bowel bulging due to the active peristalsis. (B) Submucosal tumor appearing as a round nodule, covered by slightly congested mucosa (*arrows*).

use of the mouse computer with a jog wheel for viewing certain image sequences repeatedly can be of help. On the other hand, several visual clues attest to the presence of a submucosal tumor: stretched or lobulated mucosa, bridging folds, central umbilication, surface ulcerations, villous alterations on surface, and appearance of a more congested color than the surrounding mucosa (**Fig. 27**B). For distinguishing submucosal malignant masses from innocent bulges, a smooth, protruding lesion index on capsule endoscopy has been developed[9] with the following criteria: ill-defined boundary with the surrounding mucosa, diameter larger than height, nonvisible lumen in the frames in which the lesion appears, and an image lasting less than 10 minutes. Three-dimensional reconstruction showed promising results, by enhancing the performance of novices in distinguishing masses from mucosal bulging.[10] Unfortunately, in everyday clinical practice, the aforementioned indicators are often absent, and neither has been integrated in the reading SBCE software.

DIVERTICULA

Acquired diverticula of the small bowel are pseudodiverticula that protrude through muscular gaps in the mesenteric side of the bowel wall. They may occur anywhere along the small intestine but are most commonly found in the second portion of the duodenum adjacent to the major papilla. Duodenal diverticula can attain a large size, sometimes with a typical trabecular aspect, and are usually asymptomatic (**Fig. 28**). Small bowel diverticula may be single or multiple. A small diverticular opening can be easily seen at SBCE, and in those with a larger opening, it is very common to find a septum between the mouth of the diverticulum and the bowel lumen as an apparent double lumen (**Fig. 29**), and folds radiating into the neck of the diverticulum. These features are sometimes difficult to distinguish from an acute bend in a normal loop of small bowel. The capsule may also remain for some time in the area of the diverticulum or may enter a larger diverticular pouch. Occasionally, a large vessel within a diverticulum, a potential source of bleeding, can be visualized. Acquired

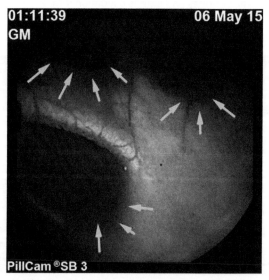

Fig. 28. Multiple duodenal diverticula. (*arrows* indicate the opening edge of the diverticula).

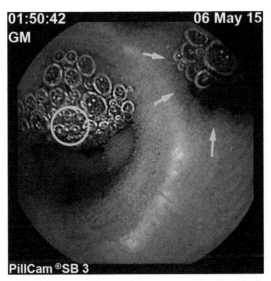

Fig. 29. An apparent double lumen due to the presence of a diverticulum (*arrows* indicate the opening edge of the diverticulum; the *circle* indicates the small bowel lumen).

diverticula are rarely found in the ileum and should be differentiated from a congenital Meckel diverticulum (**Fig. 30**), which is usually located on the antimesenteric side of the terminal ileum, 50 to 90 cm proximal to the ileocecal valve. Nevertheless, the Meckel diverticulum opening is often small, located between folds, and the lack of insufflation makes its recognition, although possible, extremely difficult by means of SBCE. A small percentage of Meckel diverticula may contain ectopic gastric mucosa or large vessels on the opening edge, which may lead to ulceration and painless intestinal bleeding.

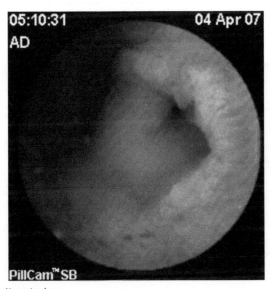

Fig. 30. Meckel's diverticulum.

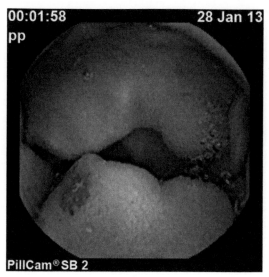

Fig. 31. Angiectasia.

RED SPOTS AND ANGIECTASIAS

SBCE is most commonly used to evaluate patients with suspected small bowel bleeding. In these patients, angiectasias are the most common lesions endoscopically identified in the small bowel and responsible for the bleeding episode.[11,12] An angiectasia is a circumscribed dilatation of the capillary vessels in the mucosa or submucosa of the GI tract. Endoscopically, angiectasias are flat or slightly raised above the mucosal surface, red in color, and usually 2 to 10 mm in size. They may be single or multiple, occur more frequently with increasing age, and may be round in contour or stellate or have sharply circumscribed fernlike margins (**Fig. 31**). When viewing SBCE studies, for any indication, the reader will also inevitably encounter mucosal abnormalities of an indeterminate nature, such as red spots (**Fig. 32**A). When

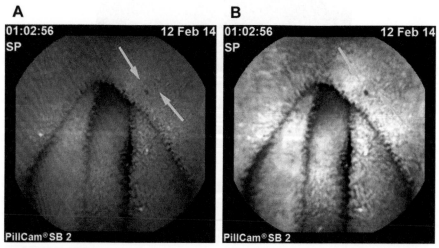

Fig. 32. White light image (*A*) and FICE image (*B*) of a red spot indicated by arrows.

encountering these abnormalities, which are often visible in a limited number of frames and may be blurred by motion artifact, the reader should report them but must avoid the temptation to label them as a definitive finding. Indeed, red spots on the intestinal mucosa should be reported as either P0 or best P1 lesions[13] because their actual bleeding potential has not been clearly established. If a single red spot is identified in a patient who previously presented with severe GI hemorrhage, many will question the clinical significance of a barely visible lesion. Virtual chromoendoscopy, such as the flexible spectral imaging color enhancement (FICE) system (**Fig. 32**B), may occasionally be helpful in classifying unclear findings that have been detected in normal viewing mode by enhancing the contrast between findings and background mucosa.[14,15]

SUMMARY

SBCE has the potential to offer a perfect overview of the small bowel mucosa and is nowadays largely used in clinical practice for diagnosis of small bowel disorders. Being a purely diagnostic modality, without the ability to allow typical maneuvers of conventional endoscopy such as probing and sampling, SBCE may pose particular issues of diagnostic interpretation, especially for those who start to use this technology. Actually, the recognition of the typical anatomic landmarks as well as the distinction of normal small bowel anatomy from abnormal findings may not be simple for the beginner. The reader of capsule images may also often encounter unfamiliar views of the normal anatomy and various artifacts that need to be recognized and distinguished from pathologic findings. Small innocent findings should not be overrated when interpreting capsule endoscopy studies, because the image acquired with SBCE is more magnified than that obtained with conventional endoscopy. Experience gained through standard endoscopy is invaluable to the interpretation of capsule examinations; however, formalized training and credentialing in reading competency are essential.

REFERENCES

1. ASGE Training Committee 2011-2012, Rajan EA, Pais SA, et al. Small-bowel endoscopy core curriculum. Gastrointest Endosc 2013;77:1–6.
2. Fernandez-Urien I, Borobio E, Elizalde I, et al. Z-line examination by the PillCam SB: prospective comparison of three ingestion protocols. World J Gastroenterol 2010;16:63–8.
3. Steinbrück I, Keuchel M, Hagenmüller F, et al. Normal small intestine. In: Keuchel M, Hagenmüller F, Tajiri H, editors. Video capsule endoscopy: a reference guide and atlas. Berlin: Springer-Verlag; 2014. p. 167–81.
4. Mergener K. Normal small bowel and normal variants of the small bowel. In: Faigel D, Cave D, editors. Capsule endoscopy. Philadelphia: Saunders; 2007. p. 61–8.
5. Koulaouzidis A, Plevris JN. Detection of the ampulla of Vater in small bowel capsule endoscopy: experience with two different systems. J Dig Dis 2012;13:621–7.
6. Friedrich K, Gehrke S, Stremmel W, et al. First clinical trial of a newly developed capsule endoscope with panoramic side view for small bowel: a pilot study. J Gastroenterol Hepatol 2013;28:1496–501.
7. Waldmann TA, Steinfeld JL, Dutcher TF, et al. The role of the gastrointestinal system in "idiopathic hypoproteinemia". Gastroenterology 1961;41:197–207.
8. Pennazio M, Keuchel M, Jensen DM, et al. Arteriovenous diseases. In: Keuchel M, Hagenmüller F, Tajiri H, editors. Video capsule endoscopy: a reference guide and atlas. Berlin: Springer-Verlag; 2014. p. 193–204.

9. Girelli CM, Porta P, Colombo E, et al. Development of a novel index to discriminate bulge from mass on small-bowel capsule endoscopy. Gastrointest Endosc 2011;74:1067–74.

10. Rondonotti E, Koulaouzidis A, Karargyris A, et al. Utility of 3-dimensional image reconstruction in the diagnosis of small-bowel masses in capsule endoscopy (with video). Gastrointest Endosc 2014;80:642–51.

11. Pennazio M, Spada C, Eliakim R, et al. Small-bowel capsule endoscopy and device-assisted enteroscopy for diagnosis and treatment of small-bowel disorders: European Society of Gastrointestinal Endoscopy (ESGE) Clinical Guideline. Endoscopy 2015;47:352–76.

12. Gerson LB, Fidler JL, Cave DR, et al. ACG Clinical Guideline: diagnosis and management of small bowel bleeding. Am J Gastroenterol 2015;110:1265–87.

13. Saurin JC, Delvaux M, Gaudin JL, et al. Diagnostic value of endoscopic capsule in patients with obscure digestive bleeding: blinded comparison with video push-enteroscopy. Endoscopy 2003;35:576–84.

14. Krystallis C, Koulaouzidis A, Douglas S, et al. Chromoendoscopy in small bowel capsule endoscopy: Blue mode or Fuji Intelligent Colour Enhancement? Dig Liver Dis 2011;43:953–7.

15. Sato Y, Sagawa T, Hirakawa M, et al. Clinical utility of capsule endoscopy with flexible spectral imaging color enhancement for diagnosis of small bowel lesions. Endosc Int Open 2014;2:E80–7.

Gastrointestinal Angiodysplasia
Diagnosis and Management

Christian S. Jackson, MD, FACG*, Richard Strong, MD, FACG

KEYWORDS

- Gastrointestinal angiodysplasia • Rebleeding • Deep enteroscopy
- Capsule endoscopy • Vascular endothelial growth factor • Anti-angiogenic therapy

KEY POINTS

- Gastrointestinal angiodysplasia (GIAD) are flat, red arborized lesions that are not to be confused with flat, red spots.
- GIAD respond to endoscopic therapy, but likely to rebleed, especially if found in the small bowel.
- Medical therapy should be considered in those patients who have multiple lesions, lesions that are inaccessible to endoscopic therapy, or are have rebled after endoscopic therapy.
- Patients who have bled from GIAD and aortic stenosis should be referred for an evaluation for aortic valve replacement.
- Biomarkers such as Ang-2 and TIE-2 may be able to predict the presence of GIAD and predict targets for future therapies.

INTRODUCTION

Gastrointestinal angiodysplasia (GIAD) is a common cause of gastrointestinal bleeding, and the most common cause of small bowel bleeding in those older than 40 years.[1] Capsule endoscopy and deep enteroscopy have increased the ability to visualize the small bowel and diagnose GIAD at a higher rate than in previous years. This review describes the pathophysiology for the development of GIAD and the current roles of endoscopic, medical, and surgical therapy in its treatment.

DEFINITION OF GASTROINTESTINAL ANGIODYSPLASIA

GIADs are pathologically dilated communications between veins and capillaries.[2] Histologically, they consist of an accumulation of ectatic, thin-walled veins, venules, and

Disclosure Statement: Medivators (C.S. Jackson); R. Strong does not have anything to disclose.
Section of Gastroenterology, VA Loma Linda Healthcare System, Division of Gastroenterology, Loma Linda University Medical Center, 111G, 11201 Benton Street, Loma Linda, CA 92357, USA
* Corresponding author.
E-mail address: gisocal1@gmail.com

capillaries lined by endothelium in the mucosa and submucosa.[3] The term GIAD was first used to describe a single or multiple, flat, arborized, nonvariceal vascular abnormality in the gastrointestinal (GI) tract, not associated with similar angiomatous lesions on the skin or in organs[4,5] (**Fig. 1**). The diagnosis of GIAD is based on the ability to distinguish them from other vascular lesions in the GI tract. The treatment of these vascular lesions is similar for endoscopy and radiography, but differs in surgical and pharmacologic approaches because of the natural history of the lesion.

LOCATION AND DIAGNOSIS OF GASTROINTESTINAL ANGIODYSPLASIA

It was once believed that GIADs were mainly found in the right colon (specifically the ascending colon and cecum) and to a lesser degree in the small bowel and stomach. Recent evidence demonstrates the opposite is true, as DeBenedet and colleagues[6] found that of 1125 patients undergoing esophagogastroduodenoscopy (EGD), capsule endoscopy (CE), and colonoscopy, 114 patients were diagnosed with small bowel GIADs. Of the 114 patients diagnosed with GIAD, 32% were diagnosed in the stomach, 50% diagnosed in the duodenum, 37% diagnosed in the jejunum, 15% diagnosed in the ileum, and 44% diagnosed in the colon. Likewise, Carey and colleagues[7] demonstrated in a retrospective study evaluating obscure GI bleeding that small bowel GIADs constituted more than 60% of the clinically significant lesions in patients who underwent CE. Bollinger and colleagues[8] found that most of these GIADs were in the proximal small bowel and throughout the GI tract. CE and deep enteroscopy has allowed for better visualization of GIADs and their presence throughout the small bowel.

Endoscopy is the primary instrument used to diagnose GIAD, followed by CE. The ability of CE for diagnosing small bowel diseases, and it superiority over small bowel radiography, push enteroscopy, computed tomography, and angiography has been accepted in clinical practice. CE can be used to target and to determine the route for other forms of deep enteroscopy before ablation therapy.[9]

CLINICAL PRESENTATION OF GASTROINTESTINAL BLEEDING

The clinical presentation of bleeding GIADs can range from occult to a life-threatening event, requiring emergent hemostatic intervention. It has been shown that at first

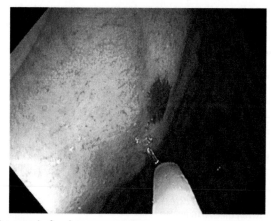

Fig. 1. GIAD of the gastric fundus.

presentation, 90% of GIADs spontaneously stop bleeding,[10] but there is a propensity for rebleeding. Reasons for rebleeding include underlying cardiac valve abnormalities, arrhythmias, left ventricular assist devices, chronic kidney disease, use of anticoagulation, cirrhosis, multiple GIADs, and prior history of the patient with respect to GIAD bleeding.[11–14] Rebleeding also may be influenced by the location of the GIAD as well. A recently published meta-analysis found the rate of rebleeding to be 34% in generalized GIAD and 45% of GIAD isolated to the small bowel.[1]

TREATMENTS

The modalities for treating bleeding GIADs include endoscopic therapies (argon plasma coagulation [APC], mechanical clip placement, multipolar electrocoagulation [MPEC], and laser photoablation), angiography with embolization, surgical resection, and pharmacologic therapy.[15] Because patients with GIADs are elderly and often have comorbidities, endoscopic therapies may not be the best initial option or the best long-term treatment strategy.[15] The presence of multiple lesions in those patients with aortic stenosis, may be recalcitrant to endoscopic therapy and need aortic valve replacement (AVR).[16]

ENDOSCOPIC THERAPY

Endoscopic therapy is an effective initial therapy for GIADs, although rebleeding rates are high, especially for small bowel GIADs. A recent meta-analysis of 623 patients with GIAD followed for a mean of 22 ± 13 months (range, 6–55 months) found a pooled recurrence rate of 34% (95% confidence interval [CI] 27%–42%).[1] A subanalysis performed for small bowel GIADs revealed that the rebleeding rate increased to 45% (95% CI 37%–52%, $I^2 = 41\%$, $P = .09$). There was no difference in the mean follow-up times for all patients with GIADs compared with those with only small bowel GIADs ($P = .5$).

Initial endoscopic therapy seems to be successful, but given that most rebleeding events occur between 1 to 2 years after therapy, this might be related to the presence of observational bias. There are reasons for higher rebleeding rates for patients who have small bowel GIADs, which include incomplete deep enteroscopy,[17–19] specifically the insertion depth of the enteroscope, as this metric determines the ability to complete GIAD eradication. Small bowel insertion depth plays a significant role in the management of GIAD, because most GIADs are multiple and hidden throughout the small bowel.[5,20] The possibility that missed GIADs play a role in rebleeding rates is very likely. Patients with recurrent small bowel bleeding or iron deficiency anemia with an initial negative capsule endoscopy have been found to have GIADs in 29% at repeat CE. This observation will lead to changes in patient management. It could be that there was an interval development of new GIADs or more likely that these lesions were missed on the initial CE.[21] Some recent reviews of endoscopic therapy for GIADs suggest that risk reduction for rebleeding rates may be little if any,[22] fitting with our previous suggestions. Another challenge in treating GIAD is that the disease course has periods of exacerbation and remissions. Half of patients will stop bleeding with long intervals between the time to the next bleeding episode[23]; thus, rebleeding may not be the best marker for the effectiveness of therapy. Some have suggested that the number of blood transfusions and hospitalizations for bleeding from GIADs may be a better endpoint. Pinho and colleagues[20] observed a decrease in the transfusion rate 1 year after endoscopic therapy, but given the natural history of GIADs, that may have been too short an observational period. The most effective therapy is still unclear, although APC is the most studied therapy (**Figs. 2** and **3**), other cauterization

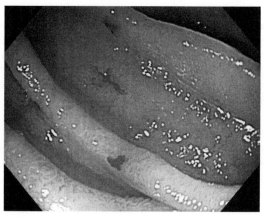

Fig. 2. Small bowel GIAD before APC therapy.

techniques (such as MPEC) and mechanical therapies (hemoclips or ligation) might be as effective or more effective in certain situations. More controlled, prospective studies are needed and will likely be forthcoming as technologies advance. Better recognition of GIAD will be important in determining the effectiveness of treatment.

Virtual chromoendoscopy used in concert with CE might enable the identification of previously unrecognized lesions, most of which are GIADs.[24] Real-time images using narrow band imaging (NBI) may provide the same effect as flexible spectral imaging color enhancement (FICE) for the precise recognition of GIAD (**Figs. 4** and **5**). In theory, it should have a similar diagnostic effect as FICE by increasing the recognition of true vascular lesions and by excluding insignificant red spots. Another potential technological advancement is the use of the Endocuff device on the push enteroscope to better visualize more of the GIADs. In personal experience, this technique enhances GIAD detection.

SUPERSELECTIVE TRANSCATHETER EMBOLIZATION

Superselective transcatheter embolization of bleeding GIAD has been shown to be successful in 80% to 90% of patients.[25–31] The most used agents are biodegradeable

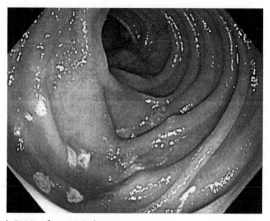

Fig. 3. Small bowel GIAD after APC therapy.

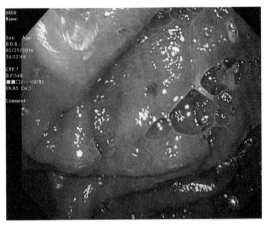

Fig. 4. Small bowel GIAD on white light.

gelatin sponges and microcoils. An advantage of this technique is that it can be repeated if rebleeding occurs. Complications occur from this technique in 5% to 9% of patients, with serious complications in fewer than 2%.[26,32] The complications include hematomas, bowel infarction, arterial dissection, thrombosis, and pseudo-aneurysms.[32]

SURGICAL THERAPY

Surgical options for GIADs include intraoperative enteroscopy (IOE) to target areas of GIADs and partial surgical resection or guided endoscopic therapy, and AVR in patients diagnosed with aortic stenosis and extensive GIADs.

There is limited published information on the IOE and GIADs other than anecdotes. Douard and colleagues[33] reported on 15 patients with GIADs post IOE and demonstrated a recurrence rate of 30% at 19 months post IOE.

An important potential factor for increased bleeding of patients with GIAD has come from the observation of the association of loss of von Willebrand factor in patients with

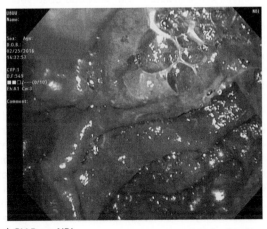

Fig. 5. Small bowel GIAD on NBI.

aortic stenosis. It has been shown that the loss of the high-molecular-weight multimers of von Willebrand factor in aortic stenosis (AS) is a cause of bleeding for those patients with GIADs.[34] King and colleagues[34] observed that 91 patients with AS had chronic anemia due to overt or obscure bleeding. Of these, 40 patients who did not undergo AVR continued to bleed. Thirty-seven patients underwent abdominal exploration, and cessation of bleeding was reported in only the 2 patients who underwent bowel resection. Of the 16 patients undergoing AVR, only 1 (6%) patient rebled after a mean follow-up of 9 years. Thompson and colleagues[35] studied 57 patients with AS and GIAD who underwent AVR. Over a median follow-up period of 4.4 years, 45 (79%) did not demonstrate rebleeding. One prospective study demonstrated that the abnormalities in von Willebrand factor multimers and platelet function revered back to normal after AVR in all patients postoperatively.[36] It seems that once these patients receive AVR, the acquired von Willebrand deficiency may be reversed secondary to restoration of high-molecular-weight multimers of von Willebrand factor, but some patients continue to manifest ongoing bleeding, despite AVR.[37]

MEDICAL THERAPY
Somatostatin Analogues

Somatostatin analogues constitute a proposed medical therapy for symptomatic GIAD.[38] There are several mechanisms for the effect of somatostatin analogues, including inhibition of angiogenesis, decreased duodenal and splanchnic blood flow, increased vascular resistance, enhanced platelet aggregation,[38–44] and reduced portal and mesenteric blood flow via inhibition of vasodilator peptides.[45] Rossini and colleagues[38] performed the first study evaluating somatostatin analogues for treatment of bleeding GIADs. A nonblinded, prospective study performed by Junquera and colleagues[46] demonstrated efficacy for octreotide in the prevention of recurrent bleeding from GIAD, and suggested continuous octreotide treatment could be effective in preventing rebleeding from GIAD. In this study, patients were treated with octreotide (50 μg/12 h) or placebo. The treatment group had significantly higher rates of valvular heart disease, coagulopathies, and anticoagulant therapy. At 1-year of follow-up, rebleeding occurred in 23% of the octreotide patients and 48% of patients on placebo ($P<.05$). At 1 and 2 years, the rebleeding free rates were significantly higher in the octreotide group (77% and 68%) when compared with the placebo group (55% and 36%).[46] These results are consistent with previous observational studies using octreotide.

Long-acting somatostatin analogues used in open-label, noncontrolled fashion have shown benefit in reducing rebleeding events and transfusion rates.[47]

Thus, after endoscopic therapy has been tried, somatostatin analogues may play a role in continued treatment for patients with multiple or inaccessible lesions.[47] It is also an alternative treatment for patients who are suboptimal candidates for deep enteroscopy or surgery.[48] The major limitation for prolonged use of somatostatin analogues is the potential for long-term side effects, including diarrhea, abdominal pain, constipation, hypothyroidism, gallstone formation, kidney stones, and pancreatic enzyme deficiency.[15] Somatostatin is a cyclic peptide secreted by D cells in the gastric and intestinal mucosa, as well as in enteric neurons and islet cells of the pancreas. The effects of somatostatin are largely inhibitory, resulting in the reduction of acid secretion, pancreatic enzyme release, and bile flow.[43] These results are encouraging, but long-term, randomized, prospective studies are needed because of the natural history of GIADs with regard to variability in remission and recurrence of bleeding alone or in conjunction with endoscopic therapy.

Antiangiogenics

GIADs are thought to arise after disruption of angiogenic pathways controlled by a number of proangiogenic or antiangiogenic factors. Vascular endothelial growth factor (VEGF) is likely a key factor in the development of sporatic colonic angiodysplasia and may play a role in the development of GIAD. It is speculated that blockage of expression of this protein may reduce or prevent the development of these vascular lesions.

Junquera and colleagues[3] demonstrated that VEGF was diffusely present on immunohistochemical staining of the endothelial lining of blood vessels in 89% of patients with colonic GIAD and colon cancer,[49] in contrast to the very limited immunoreactivity observed in the normal vasculature.[50] This has been confirmed by studies by Tan and colleagues.[51] Lee and colleagues[52] showed that unregulated VEGF expression in murine models can lead to the formation of disorganized fragile vessels that are inherently susceptible to rupture and bleeding. These findings suggest that blocking VEGF expression is a good target for medical therapy.

Thalidomide blocks VEGF expression and was used in the 1960s as an antiemetic for hyperemesis gravidarum, but was later withdrawn due to the occurrence of severe birth defects, such as phocomelia. Thalidomide has antitumor necrosis factor effects at high doses (400 mg/d), and antiangiogenic effects at lower doses (100–200 mg/d).[53] Although the optimal dosage of thalidomide in GIAD is currently not defined, it is currently used at dosages of 100 to 400 mg per day.[54]

Ge ZZ and colleagues.[54] conducted an open-label, randomized, parallel controlled study testing the efficacy of thalidomide treatment in refractory GI bleeding from vascular malformations, most of which were GIAD,[54] and concluded that thalidomide was effective in treating refractory bleeding from GIADs. Fifty-five patients with a median age of 58 years were randomized to receive thalidomide (25 mg orally 4 times daily) or iron (100 mg orally 4 times daily) for 4 months. The investigators compared bleeding rates from 1 year prior, to the rates during a 4-month treatment period, and 1 year posttreatment. The thalidomide treatment group had a 46.6% rate of cessation of bleeding as compared with 0% in the control group ($P<.001$), and the blood transfusion rate was significantly decreased from 50% to 10.7% ($P<.000$). This study measured plasma expression of VEGF and found that VEGF levels were significantly decreased from 118.24 ± 34.60 pg/mL to 58.31 ± 9.87 pg/mL ($P<.001$) in the thalidomide group. Adverse effects were noted in both the thalidomide (71%) and iron groups (33.3%), but did not reach statistical significance.

The side-effect profile of thalidomide includes teratogenicity, sedation, peripheral neuropathy (severe), thromboembolism, myelosuppression, atrial fibrillation, toxic epidermal necrolysis, and Stevens-Johnson syndrome.[52,55–57] These side effects will limit the use of thalidomide for treatment for patients with bleeding GIADs long-term. Newer biologic or pharmacologic agents that block VEGF or other components of the neovascularization cascade that are more tolerable are needed and are being developed.

Newer Therapeutic Agents

Bevacizumab (Avastin) is the most studied of the newer biologic antiangiogenic agents. This agent is a recombinant, humanized monoclonal antibody that inhibits VEGF actions by directly binding to the protein, and thereby inhibiting ligand-receptor binding and subsequent angiogenesis.[57–59] In a case series study, 3 patients with bleeding secondary to GIAD, who had failed prior endoscopic therapy, were given bevacizumab and this treatment demonstrated some benefit.[55] Patients were given 3 infusions of bevacizumab: 10 mg/kg for the first dose and 5 mg/kg for the subsequent

2 doses. At the 4.5-month follow-up, all 3 patients showed improvement in hemoglobin levels (increase of 17.6%), a decrease in transfusion numbers (61.7%), and less frequent hospitalizations.[55]

Bevacizumab is noted to have serious and sometimes fatal toxicities, such as GI perforation, delayed wound-healing, hemorrhage, arterial thromboembolic events, hypertensive crisis, nephrotic syndrome, and congestive heart failure,[59] but bevacizumab does not cause significant neuropathic complications. This drug can cross the placenta and cause severe birth malformations, because VEGF is crucial for embryonal vasculogenesis,[60] but patients with GIAD are likely not to be of childbearing age. This would suggest that this might be an effective treatment in older patients with GIAD.

Potential Treatment Targets

Biomarkers indicating the development of GIAD may be a gateway through which more optimal medical therapies for bleeding GIADs can be developed. Holleran and colleagues[61] studied expression of angiogenic factors (VEGF, endoglin, angiopoietin-1 [Ang-1], angiopoietin-2 [Ang-2], platelet-derived growth factor, and tumor necrosis factor-alpha) in patients with GIAD using serum samples and tissue biopsies. In this small study of 40 patients with GIAD and 40 controls, they demonstrated that the serum ratio of Ang-1 to Ang-2 was lower in patients with GIAD compared with controls. The same investigators found a significant difference in messenger RNA expression of Ang-1, Ang-2, and their receptor Tyrosine kinase 2 (TIE-2) in tissue containing angiodysplasia.[61] Ang-2 was elevated in GIAD tissue samples compared with control and the Ang-1/Ang-2 ratio was lower versus controls. This is the first study to suggest a link between the angiopoietin pathway and GIAD. Ang-2 and TIE-2 have been identified as clinical biomarkers for the pathogenesis of GIAD and are potential molecular targets for novel anti-GIAD therapies.[61]

SUMMARY

It was previously thought that GIADs were primarily located in the colon, but the subsequent development of CE and deep enteroscopy has shown that GIADs are much more frequently found in the small bowel. In studies that evaluated the distribution of GIAD throughout the GI tract, 75% to 95% of GIAD have been diagnosed in the upper GI tract and small bowel, 57% to 80% have been diagnosed in the small bowel, and 5% to 25% have been diagnosed in the colon.[6,8] Even though endoscopic and medical therapies are effective in the initial treatment of bleeding GIADs, long-term treatment options remain suboptimal. With the advent of deep enteroscopy, the usage of selective angiography and intraoperative endoscopy have been significantly reduced. Endoscopic therapy is associated with a high rebleeding rate and it is unclear if patients with multiple GIADs should first undergo endoscopic ablation followed by medical therapy or medical therapy first. Prospective, multicenter, randomized controlled studies evaluating initial therapies are still needed to help develop the optimal approach. At the present time, there remains uncertainty as to the best method to treat rebleeding GIAD. Scientific advances have expanded the potential for medical therapies in the treatment of bleeding GIADs, which has focused on the inhibition of VEGF, the likely next novel treatment.

REFERENCES

1. Jackson CS, Gerson LB. Management of gastrointestinal angiodysplastic lesions (GIADs): a systematic review and meta-analysis. Am J Gastroenterol 2014;109: 474–83.

2. Boley SJ, Sammartano R, Adams A, et al. On the nature and etiology of vascular ectasias of the colon. Degenerative lesions of aging. Gastroenterology 1977;72: 650–60.
3. Junquera F, Saperas E, de Torres I, et al. Increased expression of angiogenic factors in human colonic angiodysplasia. Am J Gastroenterol 1999;94:1070–6.
4. Athanasoulis CA, Galdabini JJ, Waltman AC, et al. Angiodysplasia of the colon: a cause of rectal bleeding. Cardiovasc Radiol 1977;1:3–13.
5. Foutch PG. Angiodysplasia of the gastrointestinal tract. Am J Gastroenterol 1993; 886:807–18.
6. DeBenedet AT, Saini SD, Takami M, et al. Do clinical characteristics predict the presence of small bowel angioectasias on capsule endoscopy? Dig Dis Sci 2011;56:1776–81.
7. Carey EJ, Leighton JA, Heigh RI, et al. A single-center experience of 260 consecutive patients undergoing capsule endoscopy for obscure gastrointestinal bleeding. Am J Gastroenterol 2007;102:89–95.
8. Bollinger E, Raines D, Saitta P. Distribution of bleeding gastrointestinal angioectasias in a Western population. World J Gastroenterol 2012;18(43):6235–9.
9. Teshima CW, Kuipers EJ, van Zanten SV, et al. Double balloon enteroscopy and capsule endoscopy for obscure gastrointestinal bleeding: an updated meta-analysis. J Gastroenterol Hepatol 2011;26(5):796–801.
10. Sami SS, Al-Araji SA, Ragunath K. Review article: gastrointestinal angiodysplasia-pathogenesis, diagnosis and management. Aliment Pharmacol Ther 2014;39:15–34.
11. Junquera F, Feu F, Papo M, et al. A multicenter, randomized, clinical trial of hormonal therapy in the prevention of rebleeding from gastrointestinal angiodysplasia. Gastroenterology 2001;121:1073–9.
12. Cello JP, Grendell JH. Endoscopic laser treatment for gastrointestinal vascular ectasias. Ann Intern Med 1986;104:352–4.
13. Samaha E, Rahmi G, Landi B, et al. Long-term outcome of patients treatment with double balloon enteroscopy for small bowel vascular lesions. Am J Gastroenterol 2012;107:240–6.
14. Saperas E, Videla S, Bayarri C. Risk factors for recurrence of acute gastrointestinal bleeding from angiodyplasia. Eur J Gastroenterol Hepatol 2009;21:1333–9.
15. Brown C, Subramanian V, Wilcox CM, et al. Somatostatin analogues in the treatment of recurrent bleeding from gastrointestinal vascular malformations: an overview and systematic review of prospective observational studies. Dig Dis Sci 2010;55:2129–34.
16. Cappell MS, Lebwohl O. Cessation of recurrent bleeding from gastrointestinal angiodysplasias after aortic valve replacement. Ann Intern Med 1986;105:54–7.
17. May A, Friesing-Sosnik T, Manner H, et al. Long term outcome after argon plasma coagulation of small bowel lesions using double balloon enteroscopy in patients with mid-gastrointestinal bleeding. Endoscopy 2011;43:759–65.
18. Kushnir VM, Tang M, Goodwin J, et al. Long-term outcomes after single balloon enteroscopy in patients with obscure gastrointestinal bleeding. Dig Dis Sci 2013; 58:2572–9.
19. Arakawa D, Ohmiya N, Nakamura M, et al. Outcome after enteroscopy for patients with obscure GI bleeding; diagnostic comparison between double balloon endoscopy and videocapsule endoscopy. Gastrointest Endosc 2009;69:866–74.
20. Pinho R, Ponte A, Rodrigues A, et al. Long-term rebleeding risk following endoscopic therapy of small bowel vascular lesions with device assisted enteroscopy. Eur J Gastroenterol Hepatol 2016;28:479–85.

21. Jones BH, Fleischer DE, Sharma VK, et al. Yield of repeat wireless video capsule endoscopy inpatients with obscure gastrointestinal bleeding. Am J Gastroenterol 2005;100:1058–64.

22. Romagnuolo R, Brock AS, Ranney N. Is endoscopic therapy effective for angioectasias in obscure gastrointestinal bleeding? A systematic review of the literature. J Clin Gastroenterol 2015;49:823–30.

23. Richter JM, Christensen MR, Colditz GA, et al. Natural history and efficacy of therapeutic interventions. Dig Dis Sci 1989;34:1542–6.

24. Imagawa H, Oka S, Tanaka S, et al. Improved visibility of lesions of the small intestine via capsule endoscopy with computed virtual chromoendoscopy. Gastrointest Endosc 2011;73(2):299–306.

25. Darcy M. Treatment of lower gastrointestinal bleeding: vasopressin infusion versus embolization. J Vasc Interv Radiol 2003;14:535–43.

26. Walker TG. Acute gastrointestinal hemorrhage. Tech Vasc Interv Radiol 2009;12: 80–91.

27. Kuo WT, Lee DE, Saad WE, et al. Superselective microcoil embolization for the treatment of lower gastrointestinal hemorrhage. J Vasc Interv Radiol 2003;14: 1503–9.

28. Kuo WT. Transcatheter treatment for lower gastrointestinal hemorrhage. Tech Vasc Interv Radiol 2004;7:143–50.

29. Bandi R, Shetty PC, Sharma RP, et al. Superselective arterial embolization for the treatment of lower gastrointestinal hemorrhage. J Vasc Interv Radiol 2001;12: 1399–405.

30. Patel TH, Cordts PR, Abcarian P, et al. Will transcatheter embolotherapy replace surgery in the treatment of gastrointestinal bleeding? Curr Surg 2001;58:323–7.

31. Schenker MP, Duszak R Jr, Soulen MC, et al. Upper gastrointestinal hemorrhage and transcatheter embolotherapy: clinical and technical factors impacting success and survival. J Vasc Interv Radiol 2001;12:1263–71.

32. Mirsadraee S, Tirukonda P, Nicholson A, et al. Embolization for non-variceal upper gastrointestinal tract haemorrhage: a systematic review. Clin Radiol 2011;66: 500–9.

33. Douard R, Wind P, Panis Y, et al. Intraoperative enteroscopy for diagnosis and management of unexplained gastrointestinal bleeding. Am J Surg 2000;180(3): 181–4.

34. King RM, Pluth JR, Giuliani ER. The association of unexplained gastrointestinal bleeding with calcific aortic stenosis. Ann Thorac Surg 1987;44:514–6.

35. Thompson JL, Schaff HV, Dearani JA, et al. Risk of recurrent gastrointestinal bleeding after aortic valve replacement in patients with Heyde syndrome. Thorac Cardiovasc Surg 2012;144:112–6.

36. Vincentelli A, Susen S, Le Tourneau T, et al. Acquired von Willebrand syndrome in aortic stenosis. N Engl J Med 2003;349:343–9.

37. Warkentin TE, Moore JC, Morgan DG. Aortic stenosis and bleeding gastrointestinal angiodysplasia. Is acquired von Willebrands's disease the link? Lancet 1992;340:35–7.

38. Rossini FP, Arrigoni A, Pennazio M. Octreotide in the treatment of bleeding due to angiodysplasia of the small intestine. Am J Gastroenterol 1993;88:1424–7.

39. Szilagyi A, Ghali MP. Pharmacological therapy of vascular malformations of the gastrointestinal tract. Can J Gastroenterol 2006;20:171–8.

40. Tulassay Z. Somatostatin and the gastrointestinal tract. Scand J Gastroenterol Suppl 1998;228:115–21.

41. Scarpignato C, Pelosini I. Somatostatin for upper gastrointestinal hemorrhage and pancreatic surgery. A review of its pharmacology and safety. Digestion 1999;60(Suppl 3):1–16.

42. Kubba AK, Dallal H, Haydon GH, et al. The effect of octreotide on gastroduodenal blood flow measured by laser Doppler flowmetry in rabbits and man. Am J Gastroenterol 1999;94:1077–82.

43. Lamberts SW, van der Lely AJ, de Herder WW, et al. Octreotide. N Engl J Med 1996;334:246–54.

44. Barrie R, Woltering EA, Hajarizadeh H, et al. Inhibition of angiogenesis by somatostatin and somatostatin-like compounds is structurally dependent. J Surg Res 1993;55:446–50.

45. Eriksson LS, Wahren J. Intravenous and subcutaneous administration of a long-acting somatostatin analogue: effects on glucose metabolism and splanchnic haemodynamics in healthy subjects. Eur J Clin Invest 1989;19:213–9.

46. Junquera F, Saperas E, Videla S, et al. Long-term efficacy of octreotide in the prevention of recurrent bleeding from gastrointestinal angiodysplasia. Am J Gastroenterol 2007;102:254–60.

47. Holleran G, Hall B, Breslin N, et al. Long-acting somatostatin analogues provide significant beneficial effect in patients with refractory small bowel angiodysplasia: results from a proof of concept open label mono-centre trial. United European Gastroenterol J 2016;4(1):70–6.

48. Orsi P, Guatti-Zuliani C, Okolicsanyi L. Long-acting octreotide is effective in controlling rebleeding angiodysplasia of the gastrointestinal tract. Dig Liver Dis 2001;33(4):330–4.

49. Benjamin LE, Keshet E. Conditional switching of vascular endothelial growth factor (VEGF) expression in tumors: induction of endothelial cell shedding and regression of hemangioblastoma-like vessels by VEGF withdrawal. Proc Natl Acad Sci U S A 1997;94:8761–6.

50. Kirkham SE, Lindley KJ, Elawad MA, et al. Treatment of multiple small bowel angiodysplasias causing severe life-threatening bleeding with thalidomide. J Pediatr Gastroenterol Nutr 2006;42:585–7.

51. Tan H, Chen H, Xu C, et al. Role of vascular endothelial growth factor in angiodysplasia: an interventional study with thalidomide. J Gastroenterol Hepatol 2012;27:1094–101.

52. Lee RJ, Springer ML, Blanco-Bose WE, et al. VEGF gene delivery to myocardium: deleterious effects of unregulated expression. Circulation 2000;102:898–901.

53. Bauditz J, Schachschal G, Wedel S, et al. Thalidomide for treatment of severe intestinal bleeding. Gut 2004;53:609–12.

54. Ge ZZ, Chen HM, Gao YJ, et al. Efficacy of thalidomide for refractory gastrointestinal bleeding from vascular malformation. Gastroenterology 2011;141:1629–37.e1-4.

55. Dabak V, Kuriakose P, Kamboj G, et al. A pilot study of thalidomide in recurrent GI bleeding due to angiodysplasias. Dig Dis Sci 2008;53:1632–5.

56. Bowcock SJ, Patrick HE. Lenalidomide to control gastrointestinal bleeding in hereditary haemorrhagic telangiectasia: potential implications for angiodysplasias? Br J Haematol 2009;146:220–2.

57. Baldeosingh K, Jackson C, Olafsson S. Bevacizumab as a novel treatment for gastrointestinal angioectasias. Las Vegas (NV): American College of Gastroenterology; 2012. Program No. P727; Annual Scientific Meeting Abstracts.

58. Mitchell A, Adams LA, MacQuillan G, et al. Bevacizumab reverses need for liver transplantation in hereditary hemorrhagic telangiectasia. Liver Transpl 2008;14: 210–3.
59. Buscarini E, Manfredi G, Zambelli A. Bevacizumab to treat complicated liver vascular malformations in hereditary hemorrhagic telangiectasia: a word of caution. Liver Transpl 2008;14:1685–6 [author reply: 1687–8].
60. Cohen MH, Gootenberg J, Keegan P, et al. FDA drug approval summary: bevacizumab plus FOLFOX4 as second-line treatment of colorectal cancer. Oncologist 2007;12:356–61.
61. Holleran G, Hall B, O'Regan M, et al. Expression of angiogenic factors in patients with sporadic small bowel angiodysplasia. J Clin Gastroenterol 2015;49(10): 831–6.

Inflammatory Disorders of the Small Bowel

Jonathan A. Leighton, MD*, Shabana F. Pasha, MD

KEYWORDS

- Capsule endoscopy • Deep enteroscopy • CT enterography • MR enterography
- Crohn disease • NSAID enteropathy • Celiac disease

KEY POINTS

- Capsule endoscopy, cross-sectional imaging and deep enteroscopy have a complementary role in evaluation of small bowel (SB) inflammatory disorders.
- Capsule endoscopy is recommended as the test of choice after a negative ileocolonoscopy in patients without obstructive symptoms.
- Cross-sectional imaging is preferred to capsule endoscopy for evaluation of established Crohn disease because of the higher risk for capsule retention.
- Capsule endoscopy is useful for the diagnosis of celiac disease in patients unable or unwilling to undergo standard upper endoscopy, and in evaluation of patients with refractory celiac disease.
- Deep enteroscopy is useful to obtain tissue diagnosis and perform endoscopic therapy, including balloon dilation of SB strictures and NSAID-related diaphragms, and capsule retrieval.

INTRODUCTION

Inflammatory disorders of the small bowel (SB) are common and can present in many different ways depending on the underlying cause. Many of the inflammatory disorders lead to mucosal ulceration, whereas some only cause superficial mucosal changes. As a result, patients can present with varied symptoms of abdominal pain, diarrhea, bleeding, iron deficiency anemia, malabsorption, weight loss, and/or obstruction.[1] The most common causes of SB inflammation include Crohn disease (CD), nonsteroidal antiinflammatory drug (NSAID) enteropathy, and celiac disease. Less common

Conflicts of Interest: The authors have no conflict of interest or financial involvement with this article.

Division of Gastroenterology and Hepatology, Mayo Clinic, 13400 East Shea Boulevard, Scottsdale, AZ 85259, USA

* Corresponding author.

E-mail address: leighton.jonathan@mayo.edu

causes include autoimmune enteropathy, radiation enteritis, infection (tuberculosis, yersinia), lymphoproliferative disorders, ischemia, and Behçet disease. A list of the differential diagnosis can be found in **Box 1**. This article focuses on CD, NSAID enteropathy, and celiac disease. It provides updates on the diagnosis of these diseases using capsule endoscopy (CE), deep enteroscopy, and cross-sectional imaging with computed tomography enterography (CTE) or magnetic resonance enterography (MRE).

SMALL BOWEL CROHN DISEASE

Inflammatory bowel disease consists of 2 main types: ulcerative colitis and CD. Ulcerative colitis mainly involves the colon, whereas CD can affect the entire gastrointestinal tract. Most commonly, CD involves both the terminal ileum and colon segmentally, but may involve only the SB, especially in young patients. There is no gold standard for diagnosis, which depends on a constellation of findings based on the history and physical examination, laboratory tests, endoscopy, pathology, and radiology.

CD that is isolated to the SB can be challenging to diagnose and manage. It is estimated that one-third of patients have disease confined to the SB.[2] A recent study suggests that SB involvement may occur more often than was previously thought.[3] Endoscopic skipping of the distal terminal ileum may also occur, making diagnosis by ileocolonoscopy challenging.[4] Making this even more challenging is the poor correlation between symptoms and severity of inflammation in the SB.[5] As a result, it is critically important that clinicians have the right technology to completely image the SB when inflammation is suspected. As such, a comprehensive evaluation of the SB may be indicated to make a definitive diagnosis, determine disease extent and severity, and/or evaluate for mucosal healing. The approach to patients with suspected CD is different from the approach to patients with known CD.

SUSPECTED CROHN DISEASE

In most patients with SB CD, the disease is located in the terminal ileum, and thus can be diagnosed with ileocolonoscopy, which also allows direct mucosal examination and biopsy.[6] However, in a subset of patients with isolated SB CD, or in those with sparing of the terminal ileum, it may be more difficult to make a diagnosis. Normal

---

Box 1
Differential diagnosis of small bowel inflammation

- CD
- NSAID enteropathy
- Celiac disease
- Radiation enteritis
- Infection
- Ischemia
- Autoimmune enteropathy
- Behçet disease
- Lymphoproliferative disorders

findings on ileocolonoscopy are not sufficient to exclude the diagnosis. Therefore, the indications for a more thorough evaluation of the SB in suspected CD include clinical suspicion in the absence of lesions at ileocolonoscopy, especially if there are alarm symptoms such as anemia, weight loss, abdominal pain, diarrhea, and/or extraintestinal manifestations. There is evidence to suggest that a subgroup of patients have endoscopic skipping of the terminal ileum.[4] In these situations, clinicians must consider complementary SB imaging tests, such as CE, deep enteroscopy, and cross-sectional imaging with CTE or MRE.

Evidence-based studies to date have not determined the ideal test for imaging the SB in suspected CD. Regarding CE, studies have suggested a reasonable sensitivity and specificity in the evaluation of patients with suspected CD.[7] A recent prospective study comparing CE with SB follow-through (SBFT) and ileocolonoscopy showed that CE was better than SBFT, but equivalent to ileocolonoscopy for the diagnosis of ileocecal inflammation.[8] It also showed that CE is safe and can help in diagnosis of CD when ileocolonoscopy is negative. There is also evidence that CE may be more sensitive in detecting inflammatory lesions in the proximal SB compared with CTE or MRE.[9] Cross-sectional imaging can detect transmural inflammation but superficial mucosal disease may be missed. CE offers a comprehensive evaluation of the SB mucosa. In addition, CE has a high negative predictive value for CD. The updated American Society of Gastrointestinal Endoscopy (ASGE) and European Society of Gastrointestinal Endoscopy (ESGE) guidelines on the diagnosis and treatment of SB disorders recommend CE as the initial diagnostic modality after negative ileocolonoscopy in patients without obstructive symptoms.[10,11]

The main limitation of CE is its low specificity for CD compared with ileocolonoscopy and cross-sectional imaging. NSAIDs should ideally be discontinued for at least 4 weeks before proceeding with CE.[12] An increased fecal calprotectin level may improve specificity and allow a cost-effective selection of patients to undergo CE.[13] It has been shown that a fecal calprotectin level greater than 100 μg/g may be a good predictor of positive SB CE findings, whereas CE may be avoided in patients with a level less than 100 μg/g because of a high negative predictive value (1.0).[14]

Regarding cross-sectional imaging, there is also evidence that CTE and MRE can be useful. The CTE findings most suggestive of CD include mural hyperenhancement and bowel wall thickening greater than 3 mm (**Fig. 1**).[15] In a retrospective study of 189 patients with CD, terminal ileal intubation was successful in 153 patients. Sixty-seven patients had normal ileoscopy, but 36 had active SB CD. CTE was positive in 34

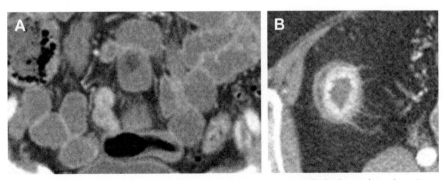

Fig. 1. (*A*) Normal CTE showing distended SB with normal wall thickness less than 3 mm without enhancement. (*B*) CTE showing abnormal wall thickening greater than 3 mm with increased enhancement consistent with CD.

patients with more proximal disease or intramural disease.[4] MRE has also been shown to correlate with colonoscopy in suspected CD.[16] In addition, there is evidence that the specificity of CTE for CD compared with CE may be better, but more studies are needed to confirm this.[17] In a study comparing CE versus CTE and MRE in patients with suspected or newly diagnosed CD, CE had significantly enhanced detection of CD in the proximal SB compared with CTE and MRE, but the clinical relevance of this is not clear.[9]

Deep enteroscopy has not been extensively studied in suspected CD but there is evidence to suggest it may be of benefit. In a meta-analysis of 11 studies involving 375 patients with suspected SB disease, CE and double balloon enteroscopy (DBE) were complementary with a diagnostic yield of 16% versus 18% respectively for inflammation, most caused by CD.[18] It was concluded that CE is still the preferred initial test because it is noninvasive and can guide the optimal route of DBE. In a study of 30 patients with suspected CD and negative ileocolonoscopy, DBE proved to be useful in making a definitive diagnosis in 24 patients (80%) and suspected findings in 6.[19] A more recent study found that DBE in suspected CD had a diagnostic yield in 33 of 38 patients (79%) and an impact on management in 33 of 43 patients (77%). Of note, it was unsuccessful in 17% and there was 1 complication.[20]

A suggested algorithm for the diagnostic work-up in suspected CD is shown in **Fig. 2**.

ESTABLISHED CROHN DISEASE

There has been a paradigm shift in treatment decisions for patients with established CD. In the past, treatment was based predominantly on the symptoms, but it is now known that symptoms are insensitive and nonspecific for bowel inflammation. As such, it is now thought that treatment based on objective markers of inflammation including mucosal healing is a better approach. Mucosal healing at 1 year has been

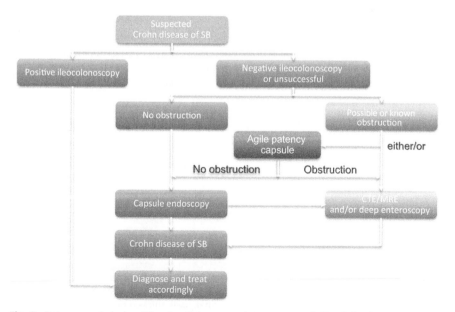

Fig. 2. Recommended algorithm for the approach to suspected CD of the SB. .

shown to be a predictor of overall disease outcome, including the need for surgery.[21] Cross-sectional imaging, CE, and deep enteroscopy are potential modalities that can help with this assessment of SB inflammation in CD.

Assessing SB inflammation in established CD is an evolving area. There continues to be some controversy about how best to assess the entire SB for inflammation. MRE and CTE have been shown to play an important role in established CD. Wall thickening and abnormal enhancement were sensitive indicators of CD, whereas abnormal T2 signal, mesenteric vascular prominence, and adenopathy were specific.[16,22] An early retrospective study evaluated 20 patients with known CD who underwent 40 CTEs interpreted by radiologists blinded to their clinical history, and found a reasonable correlation (weighted kappa of 0.57; 95% confidence interval of 0.20–0.94) between symptoms and endoscopic findings.[23] One prospective study showed that MRE and CTE are equally accurate in assessing disease activity compared with ileocolonoscopy.[24] Examples of established CD with CTE and MRE are shown in **Fig. 3**. There was a suggestion that MRE may be superior to CTE in detecting strictures and ileal wall enhancement. With regard to MRE, a validated index was developed called the Magnetic Resonance Index of Activity (MaRIA) score based on wall thickness, relative contrast enhancement, edema, and ulcers.[22] A recent prospective multicenter trial of 48 patients with active CD, comparing the MaRIA and Crohn Disease Endoscopy Index of Severity scores, showed that MRE could determine ulcer healing with 90% accuracy and endoscopic remission with 83% accuracy.[25] What is not known and needs to be determined in prospective studies is the significance of transmural inflammation compared with mucosal inflammation in terms of patient outcomes. Recent clinical guidelines recommend the use of cross-sectional imaging for established CD in addition to ileocolonoscopy for SB evaluation.[10]

The potential applications for CE in established CD include assessing for disease extent and severity, postoperative recurrence, and mucosal healing once therapy is initiated. Regarding mucosal healing, symptom assessment is a poor indicator of severity and extent of disease. Multiple studies have shown that CE can detect subtle mucosal abnormalities that may be missed by other modalities. CE can help in identifying CD missed with conventional endoscopy and evaluate extent and severity of SB involvement.[26,27] Studies have also shown that the high diagnostic yield of CE influences disease management and clinical outcomes, and thus it is thought that CE can play a role in assessing mucosal healing. In one prospective study of 28 patients with persistent symptoms, CE identified active inflammation in 82% compared with only 49% detected by ileocolonoscopy, showing an incremental yield of 33%.[26] A

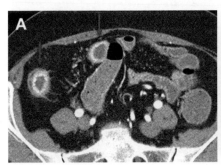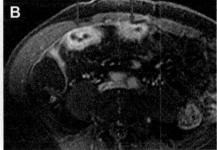

Fig. 3. Established CD on CTE (A) and MRE (B) showing increased wall thickness and increased enhancement.

study of 108 patients with established CD who underwent CE and CTE showed that 56% were noted to have jejunal ulcerations not identified on CTE, and this was the only risk factor to predict relapse.[27] Examples of established CD seen with CE are shown in **Fig. 4**. A recent study comparing CE with MRE and other biomarkers for SB mucosal healing showed that CE was highly accurate and safe compared with MRE.[28] Capsule endoscopy and MRE were compared in 19 patients with CD involving the proximal SB.[29] MRE and CE showed good correlation for the detection and localization of CD. However, MRE was inferior for the detection of superficial mucosal disease but reliably detected the presence of severe inflammatory changes within the bowel wall and beyond as well as the presence of severe stenoses. An ongoing study evaluating CE for monitoring SB CD activity suggests that the capsule correlates with ileocolonoscopy over time and that the capsule may identify more proximal inflammation.[30] In terms of future applications, a novel CD capsule is being evaluated in CD for the evaluation of the SB and colon.[31] The study showed that the

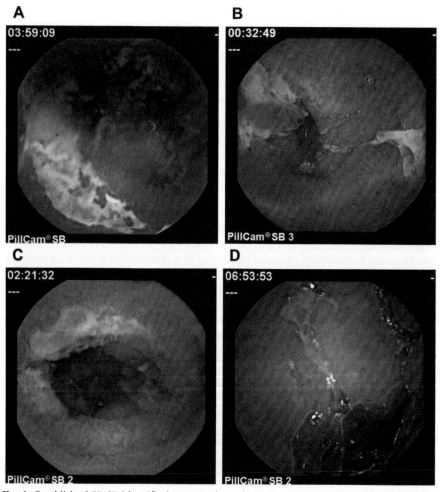

Fig. 4. Established SB CD identified on capsule endoscopy and characterized by asymmetric ulceration.

panenteric capsule was equally effective in identifying active CD in the colon and terminal ileum compared with ileocolonoscopy. In addition, the capsule identified more patients with active CD and provides imaging of the entire SB and colon in a single procedure. Another recent prospective study used the colon capsule and compared it with other modalities in the evaluation of the SB and colon in 40 pediatric patients with CD.[32] The sensitivity, specificity, positive predictive value, and negative predictive value of the colon capsule to detect SB inflammation were 90%, 94%, 95%, and 90% respectively; and for colon inflammation, they were 89%, 100%, 100%, and 91% respectively. The accuracy parameters for MRE (sensitivity 85%, specificity 89%) were lower than for the colon capsule. No serious adverse events were reported.

Using a standardized scoring system may aid in objectively tracking disease activity. For CE, a lack of a unified and standardized method of categorizing findings is considered a limitation of early adoption. Even for standard endoscopy, there is a lack of standardized nomenclature for reporting findings, disease activity, and threshold for diagnosis outside of clinical trials. Two scoring systems have been reported to date: the Capsule Endoscopy Crohn Disease Activity Index (CECDAI) and the Lewis Score. The CECDAI is based on an inflammation, extent, and stricture score and has been validated.[33] The Lewis Score is based on villous edema, mucosal ulceration, and luminal stenosis and has also been validated.[34] These scores may serve as convenient, reliable, and reproducible diagnostic and follow-up tools for use by gastroenterologists in clinical practice to assess disease activity. Studies to date have been mixed in terms of their correlation with degree of mucosal inflammation compared with other objective markers.[35,36]

Known CD is one of the highest risk factors for capsule retention, with a reported retention rate of 13%.[37,38] In a large study of 2300 CE examinations, the overall retention rate was 1.3%, with an odds ratio of 9.39 (P<.0001) in patients with known CD, compared with obscure gastrointestinal bleeding.[39] Cross-sectional imaging with CTE/MRE may therefore be the preferred modality rather than CE for evaluation of patients with known CD, because it allows evaluation for strictures and extramural findings. However, cross-sectional imaging may be inconclusive. In those patients who require CE, to document either active disease or mucosal healing, clinically significant strictures can be ruled out with a high degree of confidence using CTE/MRE or patency capsule before CE.[40]

Patients with CE retention are usually managed conservatively with medical therapy, including steroids, immunomodulators, or biologics, to reduce inflammation and facilitate passage of the capsule. Retained capsules can also be retrieved endoscopically in many patients. If the stricture is more proximal, an antegrade deep enteroscopy can be used for retrieval. If the stricture is in the distal SB, then a retrograde approach is more desirable with balloon dilation of the stricture. Patients in whom these measures are not successful may be monitored conservatively, and surgery should be reserved as the last resort, particularly if patients develop obstructive symptoms.[41–43]

In addition, deep enteroscopy may play a role in established CD, especially in determining the extent and severity of disease, as well as providing information on mucosal healing.[44] In particular, lesions identified on CE can be further evaluated and biopsied if necessary. Several studies have shown a significant role for deep enteroscopy in suspected CD.[19,20,45] These studies suggest that deep enteroscopy can play a role in diagnosis and management and may be complementary to CE and radiology. However, a complete examination may be hampered by previous surgery and active inflammation. In addition, there may be an increased risk of perforation, especially in the presence of active disease or stricture, so care must be taken.[46] If there is evidence of deep mucosal ulceration or tight strictures with ulcers that are not amenable to dilation, it is best not to proceed further.

Deep enteroscopy can also help in the therapeutic management of CD. Initial studies suggested that deep enteroscopy can help in the diagnosis and management of these patients, especially when conventional endoscopy failed.[45,47] A more recent study in known CD showed that DBE was diagnostic of CD in 34 of 43 patients (87%) with an impact on management in 33 of 43 (82%).[20] Up to 30% of patients with CD are prone to developing strictures in the gastrointestinal tract, which can lead to obstruction and abscess formation.[48] Although surgery is often indicated, endoscopy can play a role in dilating symptomatic strictures. Proximal duodenal strictures can be dilated with push enteroscopy. For CD involving the jejunum or proximal ileum, deep enteroscopy can be used for dilation of Crohn-related strictures with good therapeutic success in most patients.[49,50] A recent study showed that deep enteroscopy is preferred to MRE for identifying and treating significant strictures.[51] Deep enteroscopy can also be used for the retrieval of retained capsule endoscopes.[43]

In summary, CE provides excellent mucosal detail noninvasively for patients with CD and may identify lesions missed with conventional endoscopy. It can also evaluate extent and severity of SB involvement and assess for mucosal healing. CTE and MRE have the advantage of also being noninvasive and can assess transmural inflammation and extraintestinal lesions. Recent studies also suggest that MRE may also assess for mucosal healing. In addition, deep enteroscopy can provide even greater mucosal detail and allows for biopsy and therapeutics.

CELIAC DISEASE

Most gastroenterologists consider upper endoscopy and biopsy to be the first-line modality for investigating for celiac disease along with serology. However, there is evidence that CE may provide some benefit. Studies have shown that the CE findings consistent with celiac disease include villous atrophy, fissuring, and layering, as well as a mosaic pattern.[52] Examples of celiac disease on CE are shown in **Fig. 5**. A recent meta-analysis of 6 studies suggested an overall pooled sensitivity for CE of 89% with 95% confidence intervals of 82% to 94%. The overall pooled specificity was 95% with confidence intervals of 89% to 98%.[53] Other studies have been less impressive and the general consensus is that CE should not replace upper endoscopy and duodenal biopsies.[10]

In contrast, there is evidence that CE may be of benefit when upper endoscopy and biopsy are unable to provide a diagnosis. Such a scenario includes situations in which antibody levels are increased but the biopsy is equivocal. In a small study in which 4 patients had negative biopsies and 4 patients had a contraindication to upper endoscopy, CE was positive for celiac disease in all 8 patients.[54] There is also evidence to suggest that CE may be helpful in equivocal disease and/or nonresponsive disease.[55] The diagnostic yield of CE in refractory celiac disease has been shown to be good and may even detect lymphoma in a subgroup of patients.[56]

In summary, duodenal biopsies and serologic testing remain the gold standard for the diagnosis of celiac disease. However, CE may be an alternative to esophagogastroduodenoscopy and biopsy in selected patients who are unwilling or unable to undergo upper endoscopy. CE may also be useful in patients with nonresponsive disease and alarm symptoms and no obvious explanation on imaging. Further studies are needed to determine whether CE has a role as an initial diagnostic test for confirming atrophy in patients who have positive serology.

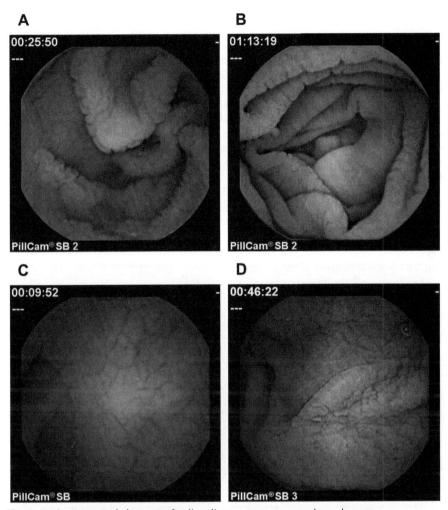

Fig. 5. Various mucosal changes of celiac disease seen on capsule endoscopy.

NONSTEROIDAL ANTIINFLAMMATORY DRUG ENTEROPATHY

NSAIDs can affect the SB in addition to the stomach and colon.[12,57–59] Although the pathognomonic lesion is the diaphragmlike stricture, it is likely that most NSAID-induced injury is subclinical. These membranous strictures, so-called diaphragms, are less common and are likely to occur after years of NSAID use. They can develop as single or multiple circumferential membranous structures.[60] One study suggested that oxicams or diclofenac were associated with an increased risk of symptomatic injury.[61] In diaphragm disease, meloxicam and cytochrome P 2C9*3 polymorphisms were risk factors. Symptoms can include iron deficiency anemia, frank bleeding from ulcers, hypoalbuminemia, malabsorption, abdominal pain, and obstruction. There have been several case reports describing this entity.[60,62] Upper endoscopy and colonoscopy with ileoscopy is often unremarkable. Barium SBFT is also usually negative. CE has been useful in identifying these lesions in patients presenting with suspected SB disease.

Capsule endoscopy is very sensitive for the detection of SB mucosal injury caused by NSAIDs and identifies such lesions in up to 68% of cases.[60,63] Typical NSAID lesions on CE show circumferential symmetric ulcerating rings usually with normal intervening mucosa. Examples of NSAID enteropathy on CE are shown in **Fig. 6**. In 41 ambulatory patients taking daily NSAIDs, SB injury was seen on CE in 71% compared with 10% of controls ($P<.001$). Five (12%) had major damage compared with none in the control group.[57] In a similar study, the incidence of SB mucosal breaks was 55% and 16% in nonselective and selective NSAID users respectively compared with 7% in controls.[12] CE is very sensitive but carries a high risk of retention. In a study of 14 patients with capsule retention out of 1000 patients, 11 were caused by NSAID enteropathy. In those cases, radiologic examinations, including SBFT and CTE, were negative.[64]

The use of cross-sectional imaging for NSAID enteropathy is less clear. Historically, NSAID enteropathy has been challenging to diagnose on cross-sectional imaging

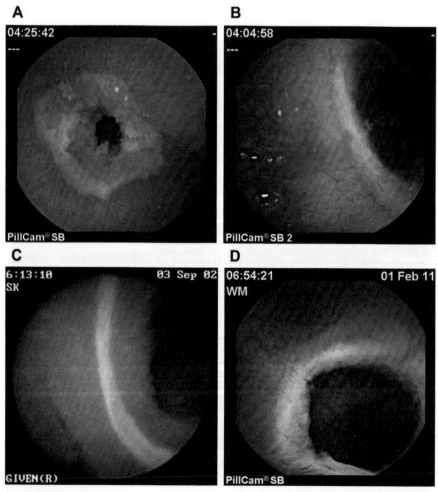

Fig. 6. NSAID enteropathy on capsule endoscopy showing diaphragms and associated circumferential ulceration.

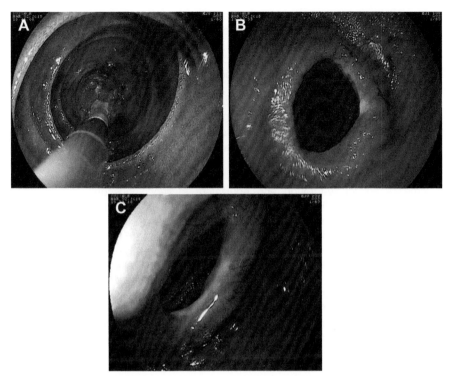

Fig. 7. NSAID enteropathy with diaphragm seen with deep enteroscopy (*A*, *B*). Balloon dilation of an NSAID diaphragm (*C*).

because it is often misinterpreted as prominent plicae circularis. However, increasing awareness has improved the diagnostic capability of imaging for NSAID enteropathy.[65] Specifically, multiphase or multisequence imaging at CTE and MRE seem to increase the diagnostic yield for strictures.

In addition, deep enteroscopy can be helpful in confirming the diagnosis of NSAID enteropathy, dilating diaphragmatic strictures, and retrieving retained capsules. Examples of NSAID enteropathy on deep enteroscopy are shown in **Fig. 7**. Because the muscularis propria is intact in NSAID-related SB diaphragms, endoscopic dilation seems to carry a low risk of perforation overall.[66]

REFERENCES

1. Chang DK, Kim JJ, Choi H, et al. Double balloon endoscopy in small intestinal Crohn's disease and other inflammatory diseases such as cryptogenic multifocal ulcerous stenosing enteritis (CMUSE). Gastrointest Endosc 2007;66(3 Suppl): S96–8.
2. Valle J, Alcantara M, Perez-Grueso MJ, et al. Clinical features of patients with negative results from traditional diagnostic work-up and Crohn's disease findings from capsule endoscopy. J Clin Gastroenterol 2006;40(8):692–6.
3. Voderholzer WA, Beinhoelzl J, Rogalla P, et al. Small bowel involvement in Crohn's disease: a prospective comparison of wireless capsule endoscopy and computed tomography enteroclysis. Gut 2005;54(3):369–73.

4. Samuel S, Bruining DH, Loftus EV Jr, et al. Endoscopic skipping of the distal terminal ileum in Crohn's disease can lead to negative results from ileocolonoscopy. Clin Gastroenterol Hepatol 2012;10(11):1253–9.

5. Leighton JA, Shen B, Baron TH, et al. ASGE guideline: endoscopy in the diagnosis and treatment of inflammatory bowel disease. Gastrointest Endosc 2006; 63(4):558–65.

6. Kornbluth A, Colombel JF, Leighton JA, et al. ICCE consensus for inflammatory bowel disease. Endoscopy 2005;37(10):1051–4.

7. Girelli CM, Porta P, Malacrida V, et al. Clinical outcome of patients examined by capsule endoscopy for suspected small bowel Crohn's disease. Dig Liver Dis 2007;39(2):148–54.

8. Leighton JA, Gralnek IM, Cohen SA, et al. Capsule endoscopy is superior to small-bowel follow-through and equivalent to ileocolonoscopy in suspected Crohn's disease. Clin Gastroenterol Hepatol 2014;12(4):609–15.

9. Jensen MD, Nathan T, Rafaelsen SR, et al. Diagnostic accuracy of capsule endoscopy for small bowel Crohn's disease is superior to that of MR enterography or CT enterography. Clin Gastroenterol Hepatol 2011;9(2):124–9.

10. Pennazio M, Spada C, Eliakim R, et al. Small-bowel capsule endoscopy and device-assisted enteroscopy for diagnosis and treatment of small-bowel disorders: European Society of Gastrointestinal Endoscopy (ESGE) clinical guideline. Endoscopy 2015;47(4):352–76.

11. American Society for Gastrointestinal Endoscopy Standards of Practice Committee, Shergill AK, Lightdale JR, et al. The role of endoscopy in inflammatory bowel disease. Gastrointest Endosc 2015;81(5):1101–21.e1-13.

12. Goldstein JL, Eisen GM, Lewis B, et al. Video capsule endoscopy to prospectively assess small bowel injury with celecoxib, naproxen plus omeprazole, and placebo. Clin Gastroenterol Hepatol 2005;3(2):133–41.

13. Hoog CM, Bark LA, Brostrom O, et al. Capsule endoscopic findings correlate with fecal calprotectin and C-reactive protein in patients with suspected small-bowel Crohn's disease. Scand J Gastroenterol 2014;49(9):1084–90.

14. Koulaouzidis A, Douglas S, Rogers MA, et al. Fecal calprotectin: a selection tool for small bowel capsule endoscopy in suspected IBD with prior negative bi-directional endoscopy. Scand J Gastroenterol 2011;46(5):561–6.

15. Bodily KD, Fletcher JG, Solem CA, et al. Crohn disease: mural attenuation and thickness at contrast-enhanced CT enterography–correlation with endoscopic and histologic findings of inflammation. Radiology 2006;238(2):505–16.

16. Grand DJ, Kampalath V, Harris A, et al. MR enterography correlates highly with colonoscopy and histology for both distal ileal and colonic Crohn's disease in 310 patients. Eur J Radiol 2012;81(5):e763–9.

17. Solem CA, Loftus EV Jr, Fletcher JG, et al. Small-bowel imaging in Crohn's disease: a prospective, blinded, 4-way comparison trial. Gastrointest Endosc 2008;68(2):255–66.

18. Pasha SF, Leighton JA, Das A, et al. Double-balloon enteroscopy and capsule endoscopy have comparable diagnostic yield in small-bowel disease: a meta-analysis. Clin Gastroenterol Hepatol 2008;6(6):671–6.

19. Jang HJ, Choi MH, Eun CS, et al. Clinical usefulness of double balloon enteroscopy in suspected Crohn's disease: the KASID multi-center trial. Hepatogastroenterology 2014;61(133):1292–6.

20. Rahman A, Ross A, Leighton JA, et al. Double-balloon enteroscopy in Crohn's disease: findings and impact on management in a multicenter retrospective study. Gastrointest Endosc 2015;82(1):102–7.

21. Froslie KF, Jahnsen J, Moum BA, et al. Mucosal healing in inflammatory bowel disease: results from a Norwegian population-based cohort. Gastroenterology 2007;133(2):412–22.
22. Rimola J, Ordas I, Rodriguez S, et al. Magnetic resonance imaging for evaluation of Crohn's disease: validation of parameters of severity and quantitative index of activity. Inflamm Bowel Dis 2011;17(8):1759–68.
23. Hara AK, Alam S, Heigh RI, et al. Using CT enterography to monitor Crohn's disease activity: a preliminary study. AJR Am J Roentgenol 2008;190(6):1512–6.
24. Fiorino G, Bonifacio C, Peyrin-Biroulet L, et al. Prospective comparison of computed tomography enterography and magnetic resonance enterography for assessment of disease activity and complications in ileocolonic Crohn's disease. Inflamm Bowel Dis 2011;17(5):1073–80.
25. Ordas I, Rimola J, Rodriguez S, et al. Accuracy of magnetic resonance enterography in assessing response to therapy and mucosal healing in patients with Crohn's disease. Gastroenterology 2014;146(2):374–82.e1.
26. Dubcenco E, Jeejeebhoy KN, Petroniene R, et al. Capsule endoscopy findings in patients with established and suspected small-bowel Crohn's disease: correlation with radiologic, endoscopic, and histologic findings. Gastrointest Endosc 2005; 62(4):538–44.
27. Flamant M, Trang C, Maillard O, et al. The prevalence and outcome of jejunal lesions visualized by small bowel capsule endoscopy in Crohn's disease. Inflamm Bowel Dis 2013;19(7):1390–6.
28. Kopylov U, Yablecovitch D, Lahat A, et al. Detection of small bowel mucosal healing and deep remission in patients with known small bowel Crohn's disease using biomarkers, capsule endoscopy, and imaging. Am J Gastroenterol 2015;110(9): 1316–23.
29. Tillack C, Seiderer J, Brand S, et al. Correlation of magnetic resonance enteroclysis (MRE) and wireless capsule endoscopy (CE) in the diagnosis of small bowel lesions in Crohn's disease. Inflamm Bowel Dis 2008;14(9):1219–28.
30. Melmed GY, Dubinsky M, Rubin D, et al. Utility of capsule endoscopy for monitoring Crohn's disease activity. Gastroenterology 2016;150(4 Suppl 1):S997.
31. Helper D, Malik P, Havranek R, et al. The novel Pillcam Crohn's disease capsule demonstrates similar diagnostic yield as ileocolonoscopy in patients with active Crohn's disease - a prospective multicenter international cohort study. United European Gastroenterol J 2014;2(1S):A19.
32. Oliva S, Cucchiara S, Civitelli F, et al. Colon capsule endoscopy compared with other modalities in the evaluation of pediatric Crohn's disease of the small bowel and colon. Gastrointest Endosc 2016;83(5):975–83.
33. Gal E, Geller A, Fraser G, et al. Assessment and validation of the new Capsule Endoscopy Crohn's Disease Activity Index (CECDAI). Dig Dis Sci 2008;53(7): 1933–7.
34. Gralnek IM, Defranchis R, Seidman E, et al. Development of a capsule endoscopy scoring index for small bowel mucosal inflammatory change. Aliment Pharmacol Ther 2008;27(2):146–54.
35. Koulaouzidis A, Douglas S, Plevris JN. Lewis score correlates more closely with fecal calprotectin than capsule endoscopy Crohn's disease activity index. Dig Dis Sci 2012;57(4):987–93.
36. Yang L, Ge ZZ, Gao YJ, et al. Assessment of Capsule Endoscopy Scoring Index, clinical disease activity, and C-reactive protein in small bowel Crohn's disease. J Gastroenterol Hepatol 2013;28(5):829–33.

37. Liao Z, Gao R, Xu C, et al. Indications and detection, completion, and retention rates of small-bowel capsule endoscopy: a systematic review. Gastrointest Endosc 2010;71(2):280–6.

38. Cheifetz AS, Kornbluth AA, Legnani P, et al. The risk of retention of the capsule endoscope in patients with known or suspected Crohn's disease. Am J Gastroenterol 2006;101(10):2218–22.

39. Hoog CM, Bark LA, Arkani J, et al. Capsule retentions and incomplete capsule endoscopy examinations: an analysis of 2300 examinations. Gastroenterol Res Pract 2012;2012:518718.

40. Yadav A, Heigh RI, Hara AK, et al. Performance of the patency capsule compared with nonenteroclysis radiologic examinations in patients with known or suspected intestinal strictures. Gastrointest Endosc 2011;74(4):834–9.

41. Cheon JH, Kim YS, Lee IS, et al. Can we predict spontaneous capsule passage after retention? A nationwide study to evaluate the incidence and clinical outcomes of capsule retention. Endoscopy 2007;39(12):1046–52.

42. Goel R, Hardman J, Gulati M, et al. Video capsule retention in inflammatory bowel disease: an unusual presentation and discussion of retrieval methods. Case Rep Gastrointest Med 2013;2013:607142.

43. Van Weyenberg SJ, Van Turenhout ST, Bouma G, et al. Double-balloon endoscopy as the primary method for small-bowel video capsule endoscope retrieval. Gastrointest Endosc 2010;71(3):535–41.

44. Calabrese C, Gionchetti P, Rizzello F, et al. Short-term treatment with infliximab in chronic refractory pouchitis and ileitis. Aliment Pharmacol Ther 2008;27(9): 759–64.

45. Mensink PB, Aktas H, Zelinkova Z, et al. Impact of double-balloon enteroscopy findings on the management of Crohn's disease. Scand J Gastroenterol 2010; 45(4):483–9.

46. Gerson LB, Tokar J, Chiorean M, et al. Complications associated with double balloon enteroscopy at nine US centers. Clin Gastroenterol Hepatol 2009;7(11): 1177–82, 1182.e1–3.

47. Manes G, Imbesi V, Ardizzone S, et al. Use of double-balloon enteroscopy in the management of patients with Crohn's disease: feasibility and diagnostic yield in a high-volume centre for inflammatory bowel disease. Surg Endosc 2009;23(12): 2790–5.

48. Cosnes J, Cattan S, Blain A, et al. Long-term evolution of disease behavior of Crohn's disease. Inflamm Bowel Dis 2002;8(4):244–50.

49. Pohl J, May A, Nachbar L, et al. Diagnostic and therapeutic yield of push-and-pull enteroscopy for symptomatic small bowel Crohn's disease strictures. Eur J Gastroenterol Hepatol 2007;19(7):529–34.

50. Despott EJ, Gupta A, Burling D, et al. Effective dilation of small-bowel strictures by double-balloon enteroscopy in patients with symptomatic Crohn's disease (with video). Gastrointest Endosc 2009;70(5):1030–6.

51. Takenaka K, Ohtsuka K, Kitazume Y, et al. Comparison of magnetic resonance and balloon enteroscopic examination of the small intestine in patients with Crohn's disease. Gastroenterology 2014;147(2):334–42.e3.

52. Culliford A, Daly J, Diamond B, et al. The value of wireless capsule endoscopy in patients with complicated celiac disease. Gastrointest Endosc 2005;62(1):55–61.

53. Rokkas T, Niv Y. The role of video capsule endoscopy in the diagnosis of celiac disease: a meta-analysis. Eur J Gastroenterol Hepatol 2012;24(3):303–8.

54. Chang MS, Rubin M, Lewis SK, et al. Diagnosing celiac disease by video capsule endoscopy (VCE) when esophagogastroduodenoscopy (EGD) and biopsy is unable to provide a diagnosis: a case series. BMC Gastroenterol 2012;12:90.
55. Kurien M, Evans KE, Aziz I, et al. Capsule endoscopy in adult celiac disease: a potential role in equivocal cases of celiac disease? Gastrointest Endosc 2013; 77(2):227–32.
56. Barret M, Malamut G, Rahmi G, et al. Diagnostic yield of capsule endoscopy in refractory celiac disease. Am J Gastroenterol 2012;107(10):1546–53.
57. Graham DY, Opekun AR, Willingham FF, et al. Visible small-intestinal mucosal injury in chronic NSAID users. Clin Gastroenterol Hepatol 2005;3(1):55–9.
58. Maiden L, Thjodleifsson B, Theodors A, et al. A quantitative analysis of NSAID-induced small bowel pathology by capsule enteroscopy. Gastroenterology 2005;128(5):1172–8.
59. Maiden L, Thjodleifsson B, Seigal A, et al. Long-term effects of nonsteroidal anti-inflammatory drugs and cyclooxygenase-2 selective agents on the small bowel: a cross-sectional capsule enteroscopy study. Clin Gastroenterol Hepatol 2007;5(9): 1040–5.
60. Deabes A, Gavin M. Obscure occult GI bleeding: an iatrogenic tale? Dig Dis Sci 2016;61(1):42–5.
61. Ishihara M, Ohmiya N, Nakamura M, et al. Risk factors of symptomatic NSAID-induced small intestinal injury and diaphragm disease. Aliment Pharmacol Ther 2014;40(5):538–47.
62. Courtenay L, Kwok A, Keshava A. Gastrointestinal: diaphragm disease: emerging cause of gastrointestinal obstruction and bleeding. J Gastroenterol Hepatol 2014; 29(2):230.
63. Tacheci I, Bradna P, Douda T, et al. NSAID-induced enteropathy in rheumatoid arthritis patients with chronic occult gastrointestinal bleeding: a prospective capsule endoscopy study. Gastroenterol Res Pract 2013;2013:268382.
64. Li F, Gurudu SR, De Petris G, et al. Retention of the capsule endoscope: a single-center experience of 1000 capsule endoscopy procedures. Gastrointest Endosc 2008;68(1):174–80.
65. Frye JM, Hansel SL, Dolan SG, et al. NSAID enteropathy: appearance at CT and MR enterography in the age of multi-modality imaging and treatment. Abdom Imaging 2015;40(5):1011–25.
66. Lim YJ, Yang CH. Non-steroidal anti-inflammatory drug-induced enteropathy. Clin Endosc 2012;45(2):138–44.

Diagnosis and Updates in Celiac Disease

Sarah Shannahan, MD[a], Daniel A. Leffler, MD, MS[b],*

KEYWORDS

- Gluten • Villous atrophy • Celiac disease • Enteropathy • Celiac sprue

KEY POINTS

- Patients who should be tested for celiac disease include those with classic gastrointestinal manifestations or those deemed at high risk based on genetic susceptibility.
- Diagnosis of celiac disease is usually initiated by serologic testing with anti-tTG, anti-DGP, or EMA and confirmed with duodenal biopsy.
- Generally, patient nonresponse to gluten-free diet is typically caused by either unintentional gluten exposure or by a secondary cause, such as inflammatory bowel disease or small intestinal bacterial overgrowth.
- Patients with refractory celiac disease may benefit from further radiologic or endoscopic evaluations including MRE, CT enterography/enteroclysis, capsule endoscopy, or device-assisted enteroscopy to evaluate for complications including ulcerative jejunoileitis or malignancy.

INTRODUCTION

Celiac disease (CD) is an autoimmune disorder induced by gluten in genetically susceptible individuals characterized by intraepithelial lymphocytosis, crypt hyperplasia, and villous atrophy of the small bowel. It is a chronic inflammatory state that heals on exclusion of gluten-containing foods from the diet. The prevalence of CD is about 1% of the general population worldwide.[1] Gluten from wheat, barley, and rye are enriched in glutamines and prolines, which undergo partial digestion in the small bowel resulting in peptide derivatives that are deamidated by tissue transglutaminase, which renders them immunogenic to those with CD.[2] Active CD can result in intestinal and extraintestinal manifestations of disease including diarrhea, weight loss, anemia, osteoporosis, arthritis, hepatitis, or malignancy. Some patients are also asymptomatic.[3]

Disclosure Statement: Consultant and/or provided research support for Alba Therapeutics, Alvine Pharmaceuticals, INOVA Diagnostics, Genzyme, Coronado Biosciences, Sidney Frank Foundation, and Pfizer (D.A. Leffler).
[a] Division of Internal Medicine, Beth Israel Deaconess Medical Center, Boston, MA, USA;
[b] Division of Gastroenterology, The Celiac Center, Beth Israel Deaconess Medical Center, 330 Brookline Avenue, Boston, MA 02215, USA
* Corresponding author.
E-mail address: dleffler@bidmc.harvard.edu

Diagnosis of CD is generally initiated through serologic testing with antitissue transglutaminase IgA antibodies (anti-tTG), gliadin-derived peptide antibodies IgA/IgG (anti-DGP), endomysial IgA antibodies (EMA), and/or antigliadin antibodies (AGA). Given the lower sensitivity and specificity of AGA tests for CD, the EMA, anti-tTG, and anti-DGP have largely replaced other serologic testing.[4] Following positive serologic testing, diagnosis should generally be confirmed by histopathologic examination of duodenal biopsies.

Generally CD is a benign disorder with a good prognosis in those patients that can adhere to a gluten-free diet. However, in those with refractory disease, complications may develop, which warrant additional testing with more advanced radiologic and endoscopic methods including magnetic resonance enterography/enteroclysis (MRE), PET/computed tomography (CT), capsule endoscopy, and device-assisted enteroscopy.[5]

PATHOGENESIS

CD develops in genetically susceptible individuals who are exposed to gluten. The clinical presentation of CD can vary greatly including the age of onset, presenting symptoms, the level of antibody titers, and a range of histopathologic findings, which can likely be explained by the interaction between genetic predisposition and environmental exposure.

Genetic Predisposition

Sibling studies in CD have demonstrated a disease concordance of about 80% in monozygotic twins and less than 20% in dizygotic twins indicating a genetic link. The major genetic determinants in CD involve the HLA, which is estimated to contribute to about 36% of the hereditability between siblings.[6–9]

HLA-DQ molecules are made up of two subunits, α and β, which are encoded by two different genes of the class II MHC molecule: HLA-DQA1 and HLA-DQB1, respectively. In CD, it has been found that 90% of patients carry the alleles DQA1*05 and DQB1*02, which make up the HLA-DQ2 heterodimer. More specifically, they tend to have the HLA-DQ2.5 variant, which involves the DQA1*05:01 and DQB1*02:01 genes in cis configuration on the DR3 haplotype.[10] This molecule has a high affinity for the peptides that are formed from incomplete digestion of gluten, which results in their presentation and resultant intestinal inflammation. HLA influence on CD susceptibility also demonstrates a dose effect. Homozygous HLA-DQ2 individuals, for example, may have an increased risk for CD and enteropathy-associated T-cell lymphoma (EATL).[11–13]

Of the 10% who have not inherited the HLA-DQ2.5 molecule (DQA1*05:01 and DQB1*02:01 alleles), most have inherited the DQA1*03 and DQB1*03:02 alleles of the HLA-DQ8 molecule.[6] In addition, there are also non-HLA genetic factors that play a role in the development of disease. In Western countries about 40% of the general population possess one or both of the HLA-DQ2/HLA-DQ8 heterodimers, yet only 1% of individuals develop CD.[6] This indicates that there must be other genetic and environmental factors that contribute to the development of disease. Through genome-wide association studies, several different non-HLA alleles associated with risk of CD have been discovered.[14] Currently there are about 40 loci outside of HLA that have been determined through genome-wide association studies that have been found to either protect or predispose to CD, although they contribute little when compared with HLA.[10]

Environmental Exposure and Trigger Factors

In addition to genetic predisposition, patients with CD need to be exposed to gluten to develop the disease. Gluten is the storage protein for the cereal grains of wheat, rye, and barley. There has been some thought that the timing of gluten introduction, the amount of gluten exposure, and breastfeeding patterns may influence the development of CD. Large amounts of gluten exposure without breastfeeding may increase the risk of future CD, although data are conflicting.[15–18] There has also been some work looking to evaluate if other factors, such as gastrointestinal infection, surgery, or certain drugs, may be the trigger for development of CD.[17,19,20]

Immunology

Gluten proteins are incompletely digested by the gastric, pancreatic, and intestinal brush border proteases. The remaining peptides pass through the epithelial barrier of the small bowel and enter the lamina propria through transcellular and paracellular mechanisms. This triggers the innate and adaptive immune response in patients with CD leading to intestinal inflammation.[15]

Gluten peptides were initially thought to activate an innate immune response. However, nongluten, proteins such as the wheat amylase-trypsin inhibitor, have been demonstrated to activate macrophages, monocytes, and dendritic cells via toll-like receptor 4, which is the receptor for bacterial lipopolysaccharide.[21] The innate response is manifested by increased expression of interleukin-15 by enterocytes, which leads to activation of intraepithelial lymphocytes (IEL) that express the natural killer T-cell receptors.[22]

The adaptive response occurs within the lamina propria, where gluten-reactive CD4$^+$ T cells recognize gluten peptides presented on HLA-DQ2.5/HLA-DQ8 molecules. This occurs because tissue transglutaminase is released by inflammatory and endothelial cells in response to mechanical irritation and inflammation. It cross-links with gluten proteins and deamidates gliadin, thereby altering the charge and conformation of gliadin peptides. These changes greatly increase the binding affinity of gliadin to HLA-DQ2 or HLA-DQ8 molecules, leading to T-cell stimulation. This activates the antigen presenting cells leading to auto antibody formation (tTG), proinflammatory cytokines including interferon-γ, and subsequent tissue injury, leading to crypt hyperplasia and villous blunting.[15,23–28]

CLINICAL FEATURES

The clinical features of CD range from classical symptoms, to nonclassical and symptomatic, to asymptomatic. Classical symptoms generally include those resulting from malabsorption including diarrhea, steatorrhea, weight loss, and growth restriction in children. Nonclassical and symptomatic patients tend to have either some gastrointestinal symptoms, such as abdominal pain or constipation, or may have extraintestinal symptoms. Age of onset of disease is at any age when there is exposure to gluten, and the presentation can vary depending on age of presentation. Children who present with CD early tend to present with more severe disease manifested as growth problems and recurrent abdominal pain, and less commonly (about 10%) with diarrhea.[15] Older teenagers and adults, however, often have subtle symptoms that may be misdiagnosed as irritable bowel syndrome.[3]

Gastrointestinal Manifestations

The classic gastrointestinal manifestations of CD result from villous atrophy in the small intestine leading to malabsorption. This leads to the development of diarrhea, steatorrhea, weight loss, and growth failure in children. Malabsorption also results in many of the common complications secondary to nutrient loss including iron-deficiency anemia, neurologic disorders from vitamin B deficiencies, and osteopenia from vitamin D deficiency.

As serologic testing has improved, more adults are being diagnosed with less severe symptoms. Many adults develop irritable bowel syndrome–type symptoms including minor gastrointestinal complaints, such as abdominal pain, bloating, constipation, or mild diarrhea. Often, however, these individuals are diagnosed because of nutritional deficiencies resulting in iron-deficiency anemia, osteoporosis, or extraintestinal manifestations as outlined next.

CD has also been linked to other gastrointestinal disorders that range from a mild increase in transaminases to liver failure, liver cancer, and pancreatic cancer.[15,21,29,30]

Extraintestinal Manifestations

In addition to expected manifestations as a result of villous atrophy, there have been many other disorders linked to CD. These include iron-deficiency anemia, neuropsychiatric disease, lymphoma, arthritis, and metabolic bone disease.[10,31–41]

Iron-deficiency anemia is commonly reported in patients with CD even in those without malaborptive or gastrointestinal symptoms. In asymptomatic patients with iron-deficiency anemia, the prevalence of CD was found to range from 2.3% to 5.0%, whereas in those individuals with gastrointestinal symptoms and iron-deficiency anemia the prevalence ranged from 10.3% to 15%.[22,42]

Neurologic or psychiatric diseases have been described in patients with CD including headache, peripheral neuropathies, ataxia, dysthymia, depression, anxiety, and epilepsy.[34–36]

CD has also been associated with the development of lymphoma. Although classically associated with the development of EATL, patients are at a greater risk of developing other types of lymphoma including intestinal and extraintestinal non-Hodgkin lymphoma. Studies have demonstrated that the standardized incidence ratio of non-Hodgkin lymphoma in patients with CD compared with the general population ranges between 2.7% and 6.3%.[22]

CD has also been linked to several different autoimmune disorders including type 1 diabetes mellitus and autoimmune thyroid disease. One study found that autoimmune diseases occurred in 14% of patients with CD compared with only 2.8% of control subjects. The risk also was found to increase with duration of gluten exposure.[43] One argument for screening patients for CD is that it may also reduce the risk of development of other disorders, although the data on this are limited.[15,44]

TRADITIONAL APPROACH TO TESTING

Based on the range of patient presentations from asymptomatic to malaborptive symptoms, and the associated intestinal and extraintestinal manifestations that may develop, it is necessary to know when and which patients to test for CD. The American College of Gastroenterology Clinical Guideline published in the *American Journal of Gastroenterology* in 2013, outlined those individuals who should be tested for CD (**Box 1**).[2]

As outlined in **Box 1**, testing should be performed on those with signs or symptoms of malabsorption including diarrhea, weight loss, or vitamin deficiencies. Given the genetic hereditability, all children and any symptomatic patients with first-degree family members with CD should be tested, and an argument can be made for also testing subclinical adults. CD should also be tested in patients with elevated serum aminotransferase levels without other cause, or in patients with autoimmune diseases, such as type 1 diabetes mellitus with symptoms or consistent laboratory findings.

Box 1
Recommendations for screening in celiac disease

1. Patients with symptoms, signs, or laboratory evidence suggestive of malabsorption, such as chronic diarrhea with weight loss, steatorrhea, postprandial abdominal pain, and bloating, should be tested for CD—strong recommendation, high level of evidence.

2. Patients with symptoms, signs, or laboratory evidence for which CD is a treatable cause should be considered for testing for CD—strong recommendation, moderate level of evidence.

3. Patients with a first-degree family member who has a confirmed diagnosis of CD should be tested if they show possible signs or symptoms or laboratory evidence of CD—strong recommendation, high level of evidence.

4. Consider testing of asymptomatic relatives with a first-degree family member who has a confirmed diagnosis of CD—conditional recommendation, high level of evidence.

5. Celiac disease should be sought among the explanations for elevated serum aminotransferase levels when no other cause is found—strong recommendation, high level of evidence.

6. Patients with type I diabetes mellitus should be tested for CD if there are any digestive symptoms, or signs, or laboratory evidence suggestive of celiac disease—strong recommendation, high level of evidence.

Data from Rubio-Tapia A, Hill ID, Kelly CP, et al; American College of Gastroenterology. ACG clinical guidelines: diagnosis and management of celiac disease. Am J Gastroenterol 2013;108(5):656–76.

Serologic Testing

Serologic testing for diagnosis should be performed on patients while on a gluten-containing diet. Noninvasive screening for CD includes serologic testing with EMA, AGA, antitissue anti-tTG, and anti-DGP. Given the lower sensitivity and specificity of AGA for CD, the EMA, anti-tTG, and anti-DGP tests have largely replaced AGA testing.[4]

Following AGA, IgA antibodies against the endomysium (EMA) of monkey esophagus was discovered as being highly sensitive and specific in the diagnosis of CD.[45] IgA EMA has been evaluated by many studies and the pooled sensitivity was found to be 97.4% with a specificity of 96.1%. However, there was some variation in sensitivity in the studies with one reporting the sensitivity as 75%. The IgA EMA can also be performed using human umbilical cord as substrate with pooled sensitivity and specificity of 90.2% and 99.6%, respectively.[22]

Further research identified the enzyme tissue transglutaminase as the autoantigen that reacts with EMA, which led to the development of enzyme-linked immunosorbent assays that detect anti-tTG.[46] Most commercial tests for IgA tTG use human-recombinant or red-cell derived tTG as a substrate with mixed-age population pooled estimates of sensitivity and specificity of 90.2% and 95.4%, respectively.

Most EMA and anti-tTG testing are IgA-based tests, and therefore a total IgA should be measured to exclude IgA deficiency. Selective IgA deficiency has a prevalence of about 1.7% to 3%[22,47] in patients with CD, which is 10 to 15 times more common than in the general population.

More recently, anti-DGP have also been studied, which are IgG- or IgA-based and can therefore be used for testing in patients with IgA-deficiency. DGP IgA and DGP IgG antibodies have been shown to have a sensitivity of 94% and specificity of 99%, and a sensitivity of 92% and 100%, respectively.[15,48]

There is continued debate to determine if noninvasive testing could be used as the only testing required for diagnosis of CD. In children the use of two separate serologic tests if positive greater than 10 times the upper limit of normal with positive genetic markers for HLA-DQ2 and HLA-DQ8 has been suggested as a possible testing algorithm, thus avoiding the need for upper endoscopy with biopsy.[49] However, 2% to 3% of people with CD have negative results in serologic tests, have low serologic titers, or have fluctuating titers, thus upper endoscopy with biopsy is still the gold standard for confirmation.

Genetic Testing

HLA genotyping in the diagnosis of CD, specifically to look for HLA-DQ2.5 and HLA-DQ8, is useful for its negative predictive value. Less than 1% of patients with CD are negative for HLA-DQ2 and HLA-DQ8.[10] The positive predictive value, however, is low because a large proportion of individuals without CD carry either HLA-DQ2.5 or HLA-D8. Specifically, the prevalence of DQ2 in the general population is around 30% to 40%, and the prevalence of DQ8 in the general population is around 5% to 10%.[10,50]

HLA genotyping has therefore been found to be helpful in patients with suspected CD who fail to respond to a gluten-free diet, to help rule out the disease. HLA typing can also be useful in patients who have self-diagnosed themselves with CD and are on a gluten-free diet at the time of presentation, because serologic testing and biopsy may be less accurate. HLA typing can also help to rule out CD in high-risk patients, such as patients with first-degree relatives with CD, thus minimizing further testing.[10]

Endoscopic Evaluation

Endoscopy with biopsies should be performed while the patient is on a gluten-free diet to make the diagnosis of CD. Upper endoscopy allows for the direct observation of gross mucosal changes of the small bowel including scalloping, reduction of villous folds, and nodularity (**Fig. 1**). Although endoscopic markers are helpful, they are not sensitive or specific and biopsy is required.[10] Chromoendoscopy using indigo carmine or methylene blue may be helpful in enhancing visualization of patchy areas for biopsy.[3]

Histopathology

Despite improved sensitivity and specificity of currently noninvasive serologic testing, the gold standard for diagnosis still remains small bowel biopsies demonstrating

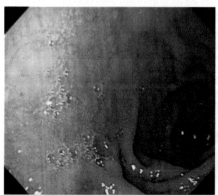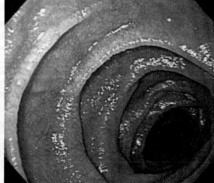

Fig.1. Diffuse villous atrophy.

increased IEL, crypt hyperplasia, and villous atrophy. A scoring system based on these findings was developed by Marsh.[51] The histologic findings can range from partial to total villous atrophy, and up to 70% of cases can demonstrate patchy findings, which can be missed on biopsy. Thus, generally multiple biopsies (at least four) of the proximal small bowel are required to make the diagnosis. These biopsies should be obtained from the proximal bowel and the duodenal bulb, because up to 13% of patients may have disease localized only to this region.[3,52]

The orientation of biopsies is also necessary to make the diagnosis. Even with proper orientation, diagnosis can still be challenging and studies have found that between 13% and 46% of cases are misdiagnosed by histology analysis. Therefore evaluation by a gastrointestinal pathologist is recommended.[3] The classic findings on well-oriented biopsies include increased IEL, especially at the villous tip with infiltration of the lamina propria with inflammatory cells, and crypt hyperplasia, and blunted or atrophic villi.[10]

Probable CD may also be diagnosed in patients found to have positive serologies and only isolated increased in IEL (>25/100 enterocytes) on histology. In these cases, a trial of the gluten-free diet with improvement of symptoms supports the diagnosis.[10]

Increased IELs and villous atrophy are not specific for CD and are seen in several other conditions including *Giardia* infection, Crohn disease, *Helicobacter pylori* infection, neoplasms, and common variable immune deficiency. Other causes must therefore be evaluated if symptoms and history are not consistent and especially if tTG is normal at diagnosis.[3,10]

An algorithm that outlines the approach to diagnosis of CD is shown in **Fig. 2**.[3]

TREATMENT WITH GLUTEN-FREE DIET

After diagnosis of CD through the measures discussed previously, a gluten-free diet with an intake of less than 10 mg of gluten per day should be initiated. Diet generally results in symptomatic improvement in most patients within 4 weeks. Generally serologic normalization of anti-tTG takes months to a year, and normalization of histologic results can take an estimated 3.8 years.[5] After initiating this diet, about 20% of patients report persistent or recurrent symptoms after diagnosis termed nonresponsive CD. The most common cause of these symptoms is gluten exposure.[53] Some hidden sources of gluten outside of the traditional wheat, rye, and barley include oats, soy sauce, certain marinades, some drug fillers, processed meats, and foods prepared in contact with gluten-containing foods.[15] Persistent symptoms may also be caused by secondary etiologies, such as irritable bowel syndrome, colon cancer, primary or secondary lactose intolerance, pancreatic insufficiency, small bowel bacterial overgrowth, or microscopic colitis.[15]

In adults, neither symptoms nor serologies are reliable to predict small intestinal damage in follow-up. Serum antibodies have poor sensitivity for persistent villous atrophy, especially 1 year or more after initiating a gluten-free diet. For these reasons, follow-up endoscopy to document healing 1 to 2 years after diagnosis should be considered.

REFRACTORY CELIAC DISEASE

Refractory CD (RCD) is characterized by duodenal atrophy and malabsorption despite confirmed adherence to gluten-free diet for greater than 12 months in the absence of other causes of villous atrophy.[1] RCD develops in about 10% of patients with nonresponsive RCD, and in about 1% of patients with CD overall.

There are two types of RCD. Type 1 RCD is usually easily treatable and prognosis is good. Treatment generally includes nutritional support and budesonide.[3] Type 2 RCD is a severe syndrome characterized by a phenotypic change in IEL and carries a poor prognosis. Five-year mortality for patients with type 2 RCD is roughly 50%.[3,5] The two factors that support a diagnosis of type 2 RCD over type 1 RCD include loss of normal surface markers CD3 and CD8 with preserved expression of intracytoplasmic CD3, and the detection of monoclonal rearrangement of the T-cell receptor chain.[15]

Individuals with type 2 RCD have a poorer prognosis and up to 70% can develop ulcerative jejunoileitis with complications secondary to protein loss (**Fig. 3**).[5] This is also considered to be a premalignant condition because up to 50% of case can result in EATL. EATL is a rare lymphoma that is strongly correlated with type 2 RCD and carries a poor prognosis with a 5-year survival about less than 20%. Patient with CD are also at about a 10 times increased risk for the development of small bowel adenocarcinoma, although risk is still low (**Fig. 4**).[3]

Therefore if a patient has persistent symptoms after initiating a gluten-free diet, further work-up should be performed to assess for secondary causes or for evidence of ongoing enteropathy. This is done through a combination of endoscopy and radiologic methods.

RADIOGRAPHIC MODALITIES IN CELIAC DISEASE
Ultrasound

Traditionally given the low cost and lack of radiation, abdominal ultrasound is the first method to investigate the small bowel in patients with persistent symptoms. Markers of CD on ultrasound include the presence of abdominal fluid, enlargement of mesenteric lymph nodes, and occasionally increased gallbladder volume.[5] After 1 year of gluten-free diet, these abnormalities can reverse. However, ultrasound is not specific or sensitive for bowel wall thickening or detection of malignancy, and therefore is less useful in diagnosing complications.

Magnetic Resonance Enterography/Enteroclysis and Computed Tomography Enterography/Enteroclysis

MRE and CT enterography/enteroclysis are useful to study the small bowel after given either oral (entergraphy) or nasoduodenal (enteroclysis) contrast agents.[5] MRE has been studied in a 2010 single-center retrospective study and although was found not to be able to distinguish between uncomplicated CD and type 1 RCD, it was useful to distinguish between uncomplicated CD/type 1 RCD and type 2 RCD. It was also found to have an overall diagnostic accuracy of 95% for the detection of small-bowel neoplasms, making it a useful tool in the work-up of complicated CD.[5,54]

CT enterography has also been studied and has been found to be useful in discriminating between CD/type 1 RCD and RCD2/EATL.[5,56] However Boudiaf and colleagues[55] only found a diagnostic yield for malignancy, specifically EATL, to be about 28%. Therefore CT enterography/enteroclysis may be preferred if attempting to distinguish only between uncomplicated CD and RCD2, given time and cost; however, MRE may be the best test if concerned for neoplasm.

Nuclear testing, such as 18F-flurodeoxyglucose PET CT has also been studied in the evaluation of the small intestine, with the main benefit observed in the evaluation of suspected neoplasms. One study has found that sensitivity approaches 100% with a specificity of 90% in detection and localization of CD-associated lymphoproliferative disorders including EATL.[5,57]

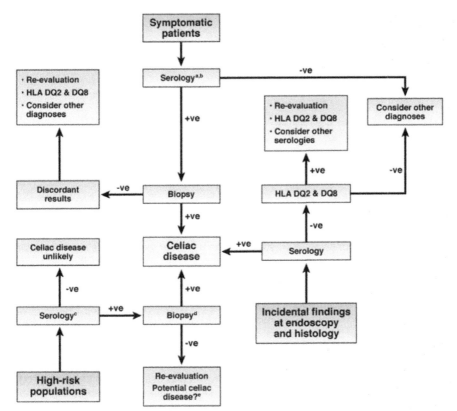

Fig. 2. Approach to celiac disease diagnosis. Serology is usually the first step in diagnosis or exclusion of celiac disease for symptomatic patients or for screening. Biopsy is important for definitive diagnosis. HLA testing is valuable in selected patients. [a] Serologic markers of celiac disease: IgA against tTG, endomysial antibody (IgA), IgG against DGD, IgA against deamidated gliadin peptide, IgG against tTG. [b] A small number of patients with celiac disease have negative results from serologic tests. Biopsies should therefore be performed if the clinical suspicion for celiac disease is high, regardless of these results. [c] Tests for HLA DQ2 and DQ8 can be performed. Negative results mean that celiac disease can be permanently excluded. However, many individuals without celiac disease are carriers of these alleles, especially those with a family history of celiac disease or related autoimmune disorder. [d] For symptomless patients, especially children, with mild increases in serologic markers of disease, biopsy analysis can be delayed, pending results from serologic tests performed at intervals of 3–6 months. [e] Potential celiac disease has been defined as a normal small intestinal mucosa with an increased risk for celiac disease based on results from serologic analysis.[1] (*From* Kelly CP, Bai JC, Liu E, et al. Advances in diagnosis and management of celiac disease. Gastroenterology 2015;148(6):1178; with permission.)

ADVANCED ENDOSCOPIC MODALITIES IN CELIAC DISEASE

Although radiologic techniques are less invasive, less time consuming, with fewer potential complications, they are limited in their ability to visualize the mucosa of the bowel and there is no ability to obtain biopsies or directly treat lesions.

Video Capsule Endoscopy

Video capsule endoscopy (VCE) is able to visualize the entire small bowel with the use of a wireless video capsule. The advantage of the capsule in evaluation of the small

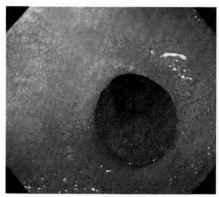
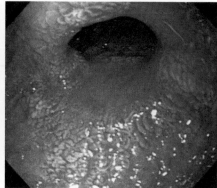

Fig. 3. Ulcerative jejunitis.

bowel is that it is a noninvasive way to evaluate a greater extent of the small intestine that cannot be reached by endoscopy otherwise. Because of the inability to evaluate histology, VCE has limited use in initial diagnosis of CD, except in those patients that refuse upper endoscopy.

However, among patients with suspected CD complication and follow-up of known RCD or persistent unexplained anemia, VCE is frequently used. Studies have demonstrated that VCE can detect mucosal abnormalities in patients with CD with known or suspected complications with an 8% to 14% detection rate for malignancy.[5] Van Weyenberg and colleagues[58] in 2013 found that proximal focal erythema or lack of progression of the capsule in the distal small bowel was associated with a poor prognosis, thus demonstrating that VCE could be helpful in risk stratification.

Contraindications to VCE include risk of capsule retention in small bowel obstruction or suspected stricturing disease. This is overcome by first using a patency capsule and cross-sectional imaging to determine if there is a stenosis, which would increase the risk of capsule retention. Overall risk of capsule retention is less than 1.5%, although most capsules eventually pass spontaneously.[5,59] Other contraindications include major abdominal surgery, swallowing disorders, pregnancy, and age younger than 2 years old.[5]

Device-Assisted Enteroscopy

Device-assisted enteroscopy involves the insertion of dedicated endoscopes into the small bowel for direct observation. This includes double-balloon enteroscopy,

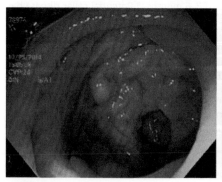
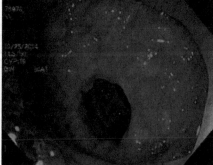

Fig. 4. Small bowel adenocarcinoma.

single-balloon enteroscopy, spiral enteroscopy, and balloon-assisted endoscopy. Double-balloon enteroscopy has been the most studied mechanism, which includes placing an inflatable balloon into the small bowel, which grips the intestinal wall allowing for progression of the endoscopy.

Until the development of device-assisted enteroscopy the only treatment of small bowel abnormalities required surgical intervention. With device-assisted enteroscopy, unlike VCE, interventions can also be performed if needed including tissue sampling, polypectomy, hemostasis, and dilation of strictures. However, this is an invasive procedure with a higher rate of complications, such as perforation and pancreatitis, which has been estimated at about 4%.[60]

Double-balloon enteroscopy has greatly improved diagnostic yield in patients with CD complications including RCD and EATL, with the diagnostic yield ranging from 25% to 33% for ulcerative jejunoileitis and from 12.5% to 24% for malignancy including small bowel adenocarcinoma and EATL.[61]

SUMMARY

In the initial diagnosis of CD, there are multiple useful modalities including serologic testing with high sensitivity and specificity, which can then be confirmed through duodenal biopsy demonstrating characteristic features of increased IEL, crypt hyperplasia, and villous atrophy. However, in complicated CD, further imaging and advanced endoscopic techniques have been studied and are useful in diagnosing associated complications including RCD, malignancies, such as small bowel lymphoma, and EATL, and diagnosing further complications, such as ulcerative jejunoileitis.

REFERENCES

1. Ludvigsson JF, Leffler DA, Bai JC, et al. The Oslo definitions for coeliac disease and related terms. Gut 2013;62(1):43–52.
2. Rubio-Tapia A, Hill ID, Kelly CP, et al, American College of Gastroenterology. ACG clinical guidelines: diagnosis and management of celiac disease. Am J Gastroenterol 2013;108(5):656–76.
3. Kelly CP, Bai JC, Liu E, et al. Advances in diagnosis and management of celiac disease. Gastroenterology 2015;148(6):1175–86.
4. Prince HE. Evaluation of the INOVA diagnostics enzyme-linked immunosorbent assay kits for measuring serum immunoglobulin G (IgG) and IgA to deamidated gliadin peptides. Clin Vaccine Immunol 2006;13(1):150–1.
5. Branchi F, Locatelli M, Tomba C, et al. Enteroscopy and radiology for the management of celiac disease complications: time for a pragmatic roadmap. Dig Liver Dis 2016;48(6):578–86.
6. Medrano LM, Dema B, López-Larios A, et al. HLA and celiac disease susceptibility: new genetic factors bring open questions about the HLA influence and gene-dosage effects. PLoS One 2012;7(10):e48403.
7. Risch N. Assessing the role of HLA-linked and unlinked determinants of disease. Am J Hum Genet 1987;40(1):1–14.
8. Petronzelli F, Bonamico M, Ferrante P, et al. Genetic contribution of the HLA region to the familial clustering of coeliac disease. Ann Hum Genet 1997;61(Pt 4):307–17.
9. Bevan S, Popat S, Braegger CP, et al. Contribution of the MHC region to the familial risk of coeliac disease. J Med Genet 1999;36(9):687–90.
10. Ludvigsson JF, Bai JC, Biagi F, et al, BSG Coeliac Disease Guidelines Development Group, British Society of Gastroenterology. Diagnosis and management of

adult coeliac disease: guidelines from the British Society of Gastroenterology. Gut 2014;63(8):1210–28.

11. Al-Toma A, Goerres MS, Meijer JW, et al. Human leukocyte antigen-DQ2 homozygosity and the development of refractory celiac disease and enteropathy-associated T-cell lymphoma. Clin Gastroenterol Hepatol 2006;4(3):315–9.

12. Pietzak MM, Schofield TC, McGinniss MJ, et al. Stratifying risk for celiac disease in a large at-risk United States population by using HLA alleles. Clin Gastroenterol Hepatol 2009;7(9):966–71.

13. Liu E, Lee HS, Aronsson CA, et al, TEDDY Study Group. Risk of pediatric celiac disease according to HLA haplotype and country. N Engl J Med 2014;371(1):42–9.

14. Dieli-Crimi R, Cénit MC, Núñez C. The genetics of celiac disease: a comprehensive review of clinical implications. J Autoimmun 2015;64:26–41.

15. Lebwohl B, Ludvigsson JF, Green PH. Celiac disease and non-celiac gluten sensitivity. BMJ 2015;351:h4347.

16. Roberts SE, Williams JG, Meddings D, et al. Perinatal risk factors and coeliac disease in children and young adults: a record linkage study. Aliment Pharmacol Ther 2009;29(2):222–31.

17. Welander A, Tjernberg AR, Montgomery SM, et al. Infectious disease and risk of later celiac disease in childhood. Pediatrics 2010;125(3):e530–6.

18. Aronsson CA, Lee HS, Liu E, et al, TEDDY STUDY GROUP. Age at gluten introduction and risk of celiac disease. Pediatrics 2015;135(2):239–45.

19. Stene LC, Honeyman MC, Hoffenberg EJ, et al. Rotavirus infection frequency and risk of celiac disease autoimmunity in early childhood: a longitudinal study. Am J Gastroenterol 2006;101(10):2333–40.

20. Riddle MS, Murray JA, Porter CK. The incidence and risk of celiac disease in a healthy US adult population. Am J Gastroenterol 2012;107(8):1248–55.

21. Volta U, De Franceschi L, Lari F, et al. Coeliac disease hidden by cryptogenic hypertransaminasaemia. Lancet 1998;352(9121):26–9.

22. Rostom A, Murray JA, Kagnoff MF. American Gastroenterological Association (AGA) Institute technical review on the diagnosis and management of celiac disease. Gastroenterology 2006;131(6):1981–2002.

23. Sollid LM. Coeliac disease: dissecting a complex inflammatory disorder. Nat Rev Immunol 2002;2(9):647–55.

24. Nilsen EM, Jahnsen FL, Lundin KE, et al. Gluten induces an intestinal cytokine response strongly dominated by interferon gamma in patients with celiac disease. Gastroenterology 1998;115(3):551–63.

25. Mohamed BM, Feighery C, Kelly J, et al. Increased protein expression of matrix metalloproteinases -1, -3, and -9 and TIMP-1 in patients with gluten-sensitive enteropathy. Dig Dis Sci 2006;51(10):1862–8.

26. Molberg O, Mcadam SN, Körner R, et al. Tissue transglutaminase selectively modifies gliadin peptides that are recognized by gut-derived T cells in celiac disease. Nat Med 1998;4(6):713–7 [Erratum appears in Nat Med 1998;4(8):974].

27. Schuppan D, Dieterich W, Riecken EO. Exposing gliadin as a tasty food for lymphocytes. Nat Med 1998;4(6):666–7.

28. van de Wal Y, Kooy Y, van Veelen P, et al. Selective deamidation by tissue transglutaminase strongly enhances gliadin-specific T cell reactivity. J Immunol 1998; 161(4):1585–8.

29. Kaukinen K, Halme L, Collin P, et al. Celiac disease in patients with severe liver disease: gluten-free diet may reverse hepatic failure. Gastroenterology 2002; 122(4):881–8.

30. Elfström P, Granath F, Ye W, et al. Low risk of gastrointestinal cancer among patients with celiac disease, inflammation, or latent celiac disease. Clin Gastroenterol Hepatol 2012;10(1):30–6.
31. Bergamaschi G, Markopoulos K, Albertini R, et al. Anemia of chronic disease and defective erythropoietin production in patients with celiac disease. Haematologica 2008;93(12):1785–91.
32. Sanders DS, Carter MJ, Hurlstone DP, et al. Association of adult coeliac disease with irritable bowel syndrome: a case-control study in patients fulfilling ROME II criteria referred to secondary care. Lancet 2001;358(9292):1504–8.
33. Hadjivassiliou M, Gibson A, Davies-Jones GA, et al. Does cryptic gluten sensitivity play a part in neurological illness? Lancet 1996;347(8998):369–71.
34. Ludvigsson JF, Olsson T, Ekbom A, et al. A population-based study of coeliac disease, neurodegenerative and neuroinflammatory diseases. Aliment Pharmacol Ther 2007;25(11):1317–27.
35. Hadjivassiliou M, Grünewald R, Sharrack B, et al. Gluten ataxia in perspective: epidemiology, genetic susceptibility and clinical characteristics. Brain 2003; 126(Pt 3):685–91.
36. Ludvigsson JF, Reutfors J, Osby U, et al. Coeliac disease and risk of mood disorders–a general population-based cohort study. J Affect Disord 2007;99(1–3): 117–26.
37. Groll A, Candy DC, Preece MA, et al. Short stature as the primary manifestation of coeliac disease. Lancet 1980;2(8204):1097–9.
38. Olmos M, Antelo M, Vazquez H, et al. Systematic review and meta-analysis of observational studies on the prevalence of fractures in coeliac disease. Dig Liver Dis 2008;40(1):46–53.
39. Ludvigsson JF, Elfström P, Broomé U, et al. Celiac disease and risk of liver disease: a general population-based study. Clin Gastroenterol Hepatol 2007;5(1): 63–9.e1.
40. Ludvigsson JF, Montgomery SM, Ekbom A. Celiac disease and risk of adverse fetal outcome: a population-based cohort study. Gastroenterology 2005;129(2):454–63.
41. West J, Logan RF, Smith CJ, et al. Malignancy and mortality in people with celiac disease: population based cohort study. BMJ 2004;329(7468):716–9.
42. Dickey W, Kenny BD, McMillan SA, et al. Gastric as well as duodenal biopsies may be useful in the investigation of iron deficiency anaemia. Scand J Gastroenterol 1997;32(5):469–72.
43. Ventura A, Magazzù G, Greco L. Duration of exposure to gluten and risk for autoimmune disorders in patients with celiac disease. SIGEP Study Group for Autoimmune Disorders in Celiac Disease. Gastroenterology 1999;117(2):297–303.
44. Aggarwal S, Lebwohl B, Green PH. Screening for celiac disease in average-risk and high-risk populations. Therap Adv Gastroenterol 2012;5(1):37–47.
45. Leffler DA, Schuppan D. Update on serologic testing in celiac disease. Am J Gastroenterol 2010;105(12):2520–4.
46. Dieterich W, Ehnis T, Bauer M, et al. Identification of tissue transglutaminase as the autoantigen of celiac disease. Nat Med 1997;3(7):797–801.
47. Cataldo F, Marino V, Bottaro G, et al. Celiac disease and selective immunoglobulin A deficiency. J Pediatr 1997;131(2):306–8.
48. Sugai E, Vázquez H, Nachman F, et al. Accuracy of testing for antibodies to synthetic gliadin-related peptides in celiac disease. Clin Gastroenterol Hepatol 2006; 4(9):1112–7.
49. Husby S, Koletzko S, Korponay-Szabó IR, et al, ESPGHAN Working Group on Coeliac Disease Diagnosis, ESPGHAN Gastroenterology Committee, European

Society for Pediatric Gastroenterology, Hepatology, and Nutrition. European Society for Pediatric Gastroenterology, Hepatology, and Nutrition guidelines for the diagnosis of coeliac disease. J Pediatr Gastroenterol Nutr 2012;54(1):136–60.

50. Abadie V, Sollid LM, Barreiro LB, et al. Integration of genetic and immunological insights into a model of celiac disease pathogenesis. Annu Rev Immunol 2011; 29:493–525.

51. Marsh MN. Gluten, major histocompatibility complex, and the small intestine. A molecular and immunobiologic approach to the spectrum of gluten sensitivity ('celiac sprue'). Gastroenterology 1992;102(1):330–54.

52. Nenna R, Pontone S, Mennini M, et al. Duodenal bulb for diagnosing adult celiac disease: much more than an optimal biopsy site. Gastrointest Endosc 2012;76(5): 1081–2.

53. Leffler DA, Dennis M, Hyett B, et al. Etiologies and predictors of diagnosis in nonresponsive celiac disease. Clin Gastroenterol Hepatol 2007;5(4):445–50.

54. Van Weyenberg SJ, Meijerink MR, Jacobs MA, et al. MR enteroclysis in the diagnosis of small-bowel neoplasms. Radiology 2010;254(3):765–73.

55. Mallant M, Hadithi M, Al-Toma AB, et al. Abdominal computed tomography in refractory coeliac disease and enteropathy associated T-cell lymphoma. World J Gastroenterol 2007;13(11):1696–700.

56. Boudiaf M, Jaff A, Soyer P, et al. Small-bowel diseases: prospective evaluation of multi-detector row helical CT enteroclysis in 107 consecutive patients. Radiology 2004;233(2):338–44.

57. Horsthuis K, Bipat S, Bennink RJ, et al. Inflammatory bowel disease diagnosed with US, MR, scintigraphy, and CT: meta-analysis of prospective studies. Radiology 2008;247(1):64–79.

58. Van Weyenberg SJ, Smits F, Jacobs MA, et al. Video capsule endoscopy in patients with nonresponsive celiac disease. J Clin Gastroenterol 2013;47(5):393–9.

59. Cheifetz AS, Kornbluth AA, Legnani P, et al. The risk of retention of the capsule endoscope in patients with known or suspected Crohn's disease. Am J Gastroenterol 2006;101(10):2218–22.

60. Mensink PB, Haringsma J, Kucharzik T, et al. Complications of double balloon enteroscopy: a multicenter survey. Endoscopy 2007;39(7):613–5.

61. Hadithi M, Al-toma A, Oudejans J, et al. The value of double-balloon enteroscopy in patients with refractory celiac disease. Am J Gastroenterol 2007;102(5): 987–96.

Neoplastic Diseases of the Small Bowel

Emanuele Rondonotti, MD, PhD[a],*, Anastasios Koulaouzidis, MD, FRCPE[b],
Diana E. Yung, MBChB[b], Surekha N. Reddy, MBChB, MRCS, MD, FRCR[c],
Julius Georgiou, DIC, MEng, ACGI, SMIEEE[d], Marco Pennazio, MD[e]

KEYWORDS

- Small bowel tumors • Capsule endoscopy • Device-assisted enteroscopy
- CT-enteroclysis • MR-enteroclysis • CT enterography • MR enterography

KEY POINTS

- The incidence of small bowel tumors is increasing over time.
- Due to its ability to inspect the entire small bowel in a noninvasive manner, capsule endoscopy (CE) is an ideal diagnostic tool when a nonobstructing small bowel tumor is suspected.
- Dedicated small bowel cross-sectional imaging techniques have a key role in both diagnosis and preoperative staging of small bowel tumors.
- Device-assisted enteroscopy (DAE) provides definitive diagnosis by allowing collection of tissue samples; moreover, by marking the identified lesion, it enables its easier recognition at time of surgery.
- In the diagnostic work-up of small bowel tumors, CE, DAE, and advanced radiologic imaging techniques are complementary rather than competing modalities.

Disclosure Statements: All the authors do not declare any commercial or financial conflict of interest and any funding sources related to this work.
Author Contribution: E. Rondonotti, D.E. Yung, S.N. Reddy, J. Georgoiu, and A. Koulaouzids substantially contributed to the article conception and drafted the article; M. Pennazio supervised the work and revised it critically for important intellectual content. All the authors approved the final version to be published.
[a] Gastroenterology Unit, Valduce Hospital, Via Dante 11, Como 22100, Italy; [b] Centre for Liver & Digestive Disorders, The Royal Infirmary of Edinburgh, Edinburgh EH16 4SA, UK; [c] Department of Radiology, Western General Hospital, Crewe Road South, 51 Little France Crescent, Edinburgh EH3 9JD, UK; [d] Department of Electrical and Computer Engineering, University of Cyprus, Cyprus 1 University Avenue, Aglantzia 2109, Cyprus; [e] Division of Gastroenterology U, San Giovanni AS University-Teaching Hospital, Via Cavour 31, Torino 10123, Italy
* Corresponding author. Gastroenterology Unit, Valduce Hospital, Via Dante 10, Como 22100, Italy.
E-mail address: ema.rondo@gmail.com

giendo.theclinics.com

INTRODUCTION

Although the small bowel represents 75% of the length and 90% of the overall mucosal surface of the gastrointestinal (GI) tract, it is a rare location for the development of neoplasms. Overall, small bowel tumors account for 3% to 6% of all GI neoplasms and 1% to 3% of all GI malignancies.[1–3] Despite the identification of more than 40 different histologic types of small intestinal tumors,[4,5] there are 4 major histologic subtypes: approximately 30% to 45% of small bowel tumors are adenocarcinomas, 20% to 40% neuroendocrine tumors, 10% to 20% lymphomas, and 10% to 15% sarcomas.[5,6]

According to the US Surveillance, Epidemiology, and End Results (SEER) program, the rate of new cases, age-adjusted and based on 2009 to 2013 diagnoses, is 2.2 per 100,000 persons per year.[7] Therefore, it is estimated that in 2016 approximately 10,000 people in the United States will be diagnosed with small intestinal cancer and approximately 1300 people will die of it.[7] International data show that the incidence varies across countries, higher in Western counties and Oceania than in Asia, with an incidence ratio of 2 to 2.5 when US and Japanese populations are compared.[1,8–14] A higher incidence rate is observed in the black US population compared with whites,[7,15] and a high incidence rate is also reported among the Maori of New Zealand (approximately 4 cases per 100.000 per year) and Hawaiians.[1] In most countries, the overall incidence of small bowel tumors is higher in men than in women; it starts increasing after the age of 40 to 45 years and tends to rise with age, until the age of 75. The median age at diagnosis is approximately 65 years.[1,4–6,16–19]

Although some differences exist among studies, mostly concerning the incidence patterns of specific histologic subtypes, several studies consistently show an increasing overall incidence rate of small bowel neoplasms over time. The US SEER program[7] reported that over the past 20 years (from 1992 to 2013) it increased from 1.5 to 2.2 cases per 100,000 inhabitants (**Fig. 1**). It is, therefore, calculated that rates for new small bowel cancer cases have been rising on average 2.4% each year over the past 10 years.[7] Similar time-trend figures were also reported in recent studies from European countries, such as the United Kingdom,[16] Sweden,[17] France,[18] and Denmark.[19] Currently, the reason for this increase remains largely unexplained. Taking into account the epidemiologic trends of predisposing diseases (ie, celiac disease and

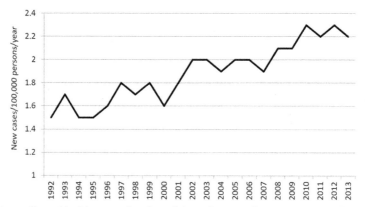

Fig. 1. Age-adjusted incidence ratio of small bowel tumors between 1992 and 2013 in the Untied States based on SEER program. (*Modified from* National Cancer Institute. SEER stat fact sheets: small intestine cancer. Available at: http://seer.cancer.gov/statfacts/html/smint.html. Accessed 25 March, 2016.)

inflammatory bowel diseases),[5] however, the behavioral and environmental risk factors associated with small bowel tumors (ie, obesity[5,8,20,21] and cigarette smoking[5,22–24]) and the aging of populations, this trend is likely to continue, and small intestinal cancer is likely to become an increasing part of the gastroenterological workload in the next few years.

Despite obvious differences among histologic subtypes, currently, the overall prognosis of small bowel tumors remains poor. Whereas cancers at other sites have increasing long-term survival rates over the past 2 decades, the US data from 1985 to 2000 showed no significant change in long-term survival rates for any of the 4 main histologic subtypes of small bowel tumors.[7] Consistently, Lepage and colleagues[18] showed no significant improvement in the survival rate over a 26-year period (1989–2001). Concerning small bowel tumors, earlier tumor stages at diagnosis (stage I and II), small tumor size, and curative resection have been identified as factors favoring overall survival. Conversely, poorly differentiated tumors, lymph node involvement, and distant metastases are the main factors predicting poorer prognosis.[7,17–19,25–27] A majority of these factors largely depend on the timing of diagnosis, which is often delayed (delays of 3 years for benign tumors and 1.5 years for malignant tumors have been estimated).[6] Some specific features of small bowel tumors, which grow slowly and extraluminally, remaining asymptomatic for years or presenting with nonspecific complaints, can contribute in delaying the diagnosis. Nevertheless, at least until recently, the technical difficulties in exploring the small bowel were one of the most important barriers in reaching a timely and definite diagnosis. Recent data suggest that the introduction of diagnostic techniques specifically dedicated to evaluation of the small bowel as well as new drugs for the treatment of specific histologic subtypes of tumors (ie, imatinib and sunitinib for GI stromal tumors [GISTs])[28,29] may change these figures. A recent study[30] reported a shift in the diagnostic process of patients with small bowel tumors, with an increasing number of patients being diagnosed through CE. Consistently, a study from Portugal[31] showed that in the time frame 2010 to 2014, more than 50% of patients diagnosed with small bowel tumors received the diagnosis by endoscopy or imaging techniques whereas only 24% of them received the final diagnosis at time of surgery. Moreover, Honda and colleagues[32] underlined that in the time frame 2003 to 2011, when deep enteroscopy techniques were readily available, the median diagnostic delay was shorter than previously reported, 4.3 months for small bowel tumors overall and 4.9 months and 3.6 months for benign and malignant tumors, respectively. Consequently, an increased rate of patients received elective surgical intervention, instead of undergoing surgery for acute abdomen due to obstructive symptoms. Furthermore, the SEER program reported encouraging data: focusing on recent trends (2004–2013), despite the increasing incidence of small bowel tumors, the mortality rate has remained stable and an increasing overall 5-year survival rate has been observed.[7] Similarly, according to EUROCARE-5 data, overall 5-year survival increased from 40.5% (1999–2001) to 48.7% (2005–2007).[33]

The available evidence on the role of new tools in the diagnosis and management of small bowel tumors is reviewed, highlighting their strengths and limitations and how their combined use can possibly contribute in modifying both detection and prognosis of small bowel neoplasms.

SMALL BOWEL CAPSULE ENDOSCOPY

The detection rate of small bowel tumors via CE ranges from 1.5% to 9%[34,35] and from 3% to 5% in studies collecting more than 1000 patients.[36–39] The rate of small bowel tumors has increased in patients undergoing CE for obscure GI bleeding.[36–38] Among them, the detection of tumors is higher in those presenting with obscure-overt bleeding and in those under the age of 50. Although vascular lesions are the most common finding in older patients, in younger patients, small bowel CE often identifies inflammatory or neoplastic changes.[40] These data contributed to raise awareness of the importance of prioritizing small bowel evaluation in young patients with obscure GI bleeding. Moreover, CE is perceived as a noninvasive test and it is better tolerated than other diagnostic methods for the study of the small bowel, mainly compared with DAE.[41] Furthermore, CE offers the opportunity of a detailed and panoramic view of the entire small bowel. For all these reasons, CE often represents the first diagnostic test performed in patients with small bowel tumors.

Nevertheless, in a large retrospective study of more than 690 patients, Lewis and colleagues[42] calculated that the CE miss rate for neoplasms was 18.9%. In the same study, however, the miss rates for vascular lesions and ulcers were 5.9% and 0.5%, respectively. Several studies have recently reported cases of small bowel tumors missed by CE and identified by means of DAE and/or dedicated small bowel cross-sectional imaging techniques.[43,44] CE can miss neoplastic lesions because of limited visualization in the setting of poor bowel preparation, which occurs in approximately 10% to 15% of examinations, regardless of preparation regimen.[45] In addition, the capsule is passively propelled by natural peristalsis, which can lead to quick capsule transit, mostly in the distal duodenum and proximal jejunum, where 25% to 30% of small bowel tumors are located. Small bowel motility studies have revealed that short bursts of a very fast movement (>15 cm/min) occur for approximately 45 minutes after pyloric passage, probably reflecting phase III of the migrating motor complex.[46] Furthermore, it has been demonstrated that the sensitivity of CE in identifying glass beads sewn into the intestine of dogs is inferior to that of push enteroscopy (64% and 37%, respectively).[47] Honda and colleagues[32] found that the diagnostic yield of CE for small bowel tumors located in the proximal small bowel is significantly lower than that observed for small bowel tumors located in the distal small bowel (73% vs 90%; $P = .040$). Therefore, the visualization of the ampulla of Vater during the examination (which indicate an adequate proximal small bowel examination) should be considered a CE key quality indicator.[48] In this regard, a recently developed capsule with a 360° lateral panoramic showed promising results.[49]

Even when focusing the attention on the lower end of the small bowel (Hatzaras and colleagues[13] reported that up to 30% of small bowel tumors are located in the distal small bowel), CE can miss neoplastic lesions mostly because the quality of small bowel preparation seems to decrease along the small bowel.[50] Additionally, the capsule does not reach the ileocecal valve during recording time in approximately 15% to 20% of cases.[51] Theoretically, prokinetic agents can be used to shorten the gastric transit time to improve completion rate. Therefore, various prokinetics (ie, erythromycin, mosapride, metoclopramide, and lubiprostone) have been investigated for bowel preparation of CE.[52] Nevertheless, adding prokinetic agents to the bowel preparation does not seem to enhance either the completion rate or the diagnostic yield. Therefore, routine prokinetic administration is not recommended.[53,54] Conversely, the targeted administration of a prokinetic, based on the systematic and repeated checking of capsule position through a real-time viewer, seems to significantly increase the rate of complete enteroscopy.[55]

The passive uncontrollable capsule movement poses significant difficulty in differentiating a real submucosal mass from innocent mucosal bulges. Up to half of all small bowel malignancies, such as GISTs and neuroendocrine tumors (**Fig. 2**), arise from the submucosal layer of the intestinal wall[56]; hence, they appear as bulges with certain

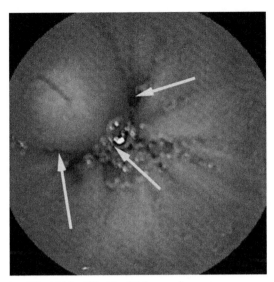

Fig. 2. Small bowel carcinoid identified by CE (*arrows*).

surface morphologic characteristics. Girelli and colleagues[56] attempted to devise and validate an index based on these characteristics (smooth, protruding lesion index on CE [SPICE]) to discriminate submucosal masses from innocent bulges. Although SPICE presents favorable diagnostic accuracy, it has not yet been incorporated into any proprietary reviewing software. Shyung and colleagues[57] described a scoring system to interpret CE findings in small bowel tumors. The proposed tumor score comprises 5 components: bleeding, mucosal disruption, irregular surface, color, and white villi. These can be scored for probability of mass lesions seen at CE.[57] To that end, it has also been shown that applying 3-D reconstruction to the standard 2-D video reading platform does not improve the performance of expert small bowel capsule endoscopy readers, although it significantly increases the performance of novices in distinguishing masses from bulges.[58]

Although capsule retention occurs in an estimated 2% of all patients undergoing this examination,[51] small bowel tumors are one of the major diseases associated with this complication. Taking into account that the retention is generally asymptomatic and most patients with a small bowel tumor undergo surgical resection (with the possibility of easy retrieval of a capsule), however, in cases of suspected small bowel tumor, patency investigation before CE is still not recommended by current guidelines.[59]

In light of the limitations of CE in the specific setting of small bowel tumors, several technical developments have been trialed to improve the capability of the device in identifying and classifying small bowel tumors. Recently, Fuji Intelligent Chromo Endoscopy (FICE), a spectral estimation technology based on arithmetical processing of ordinary images (Fujinon. Tokyo, Japan) that is integrated into proprietary software, has been tested. Unfortunately, it does not seem to improve the visualization of small bowel tumors.[60] Augmented Live-Body Image Color-Spectrum Enhancement (ALICE), another spectral imaging technique for the MiroView system (IntroMedic, Seoul, Korea), has shown limited and equally disappointing data.[61] Infrared fluorescence endoscopy, in conjunction with an infrared fluorescent-labeling contrast agent, is a well-known technique used for efficient early stage cancer detection. There is currently a screening capsule prototype (**Fig. 3**), which is able to detect infrared

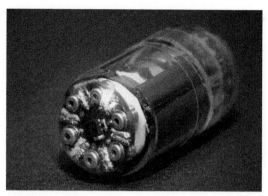

Fig. 3. Prototype of the infrared fluorescence-based cancer screening capsule for the small bowel.

fluorescence emitted by indocyanine green (ICG) fluorophore dye. Rather than images, the capsule works as a high-sensitivity fluorometer that records fluorescence levels throughout the small intestine. Ex vivo experiments on ICG-impregnated swine intestine have shown that the prototype system is able to detect low concentrations of ICG in the nanomolar and micromolar regions. This could prove useful in detecting early cancer in the small bowel.[62] Hyperspectral imaging is emerging as another promising technology for medical diagnosis. Hyperspectral images present large amounts of information from the mucosal surface, which are captured by sensors. Using this information and a set of complex classification algorithms, it is possible to determine the material or substance located at each pixel. This technique has been used by neurosurgeons in the process of brain tumor resection, avoiding the excessive extraction of normal tissue and unintentionally leaving small remnants of tumor. Such precise delineation of tumor boundaries improves the results of surgery. Preliminary results indicate that it is possible to discriminate between healthy and tumor tissues in the brain by exclusively processing the spectral information of the tissues.[63,64]

DEDICATED SMALL BOWEL CROSS-SECTIONAL RADIOLOGIC IMAGING

Small bowel barium follow-through studies were once the mainstay of small bowel imaging, but these have now largely been superseded by dedicated small bowel cross-sectional imaging techniques, namely magnetic resonance (MR) and CT.[59] Because collapsed bowel loops can hide lesions or may mimic small bowel diseases, both techniques require luminal distension of the intestinal loops to identify small bowel lesions. This is achieved by administering luminal contrast agents.

Two types of oral contrast agents can be used for CT: positive and neutral. The former (**Fig. 4**) provides an excellent background, facilitating detection of lesions protruding into the lumen and identification of mucosal details. It can hamper the detailed evaluation of mural features, however, when intravenous contrast is administered. Conversely, the latter (neutral or near-water attenuation contrast agent) (**Fig. 5**) allows depiction of mucosal folds and assessment of mucosal enhancement and provides optimal bowel dilation.[65] Oral contrast media for MR can be classified as positive, negative, or biphasic, according to the signal intensity of bowel lumen. With positive paramagnetic compounds (ie, water-based gadolinium solutions), the lumen signal is high (it appears as white), potentially masking the wall enhancement obtained by intravenous gadolinium administration. Negative contrast agents are

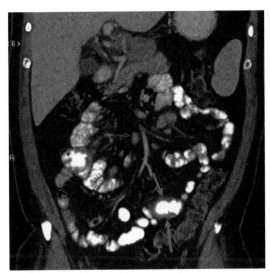

Fig. 4. Coronal CT enterography image with positive oral contrast demonstrates a short segment of proximal ileal thickening (*red arrows*) due to small bowel lymphoma, with low-volume but size-significant mesenteric nodes (*blue arrows*).

superparamagnetic (ie, water-based solutions of iron oxide particles coated with silicone) and produce low-signal intensity (the lumen appears dark), allowing better visualization of the bowel wall and mesenteric fat. Finally, biphasic contrast agents (aqueous solutions of hyperosmotic compounds [ie, polyethylene glycol]) produce both the positive effect on T2-weighted sequences and the dark lumen appearance on T1-weighted sequences; therefore, they are the most versatile agents, which are frequently used when small bowel tumors are suspected.[66,67]

For both CT and MR, luminal contrast agents can be administered either orally (enterography) or through a nasojejunal tube (enteroclysis). Enteroclysis may offer better bowel distension (the contrast is infused by means of a pressure-controlled electric pump at a

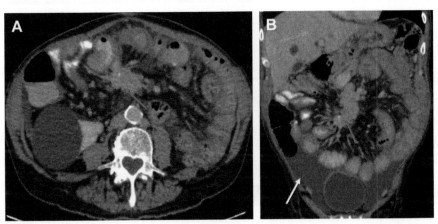

Fig. 5. CT enterography axial (*A*) and coronal (*B*) images demonstrate a carcinoid mass within the small bowel mesentery (*red arrows*) with flecks of calcification; white arrow shows pelvic ascites.

rate of 100–160 mL/min), but it requires nasojejunal tube placement beyond the ligament of Treitz. On the other hand, enterography is better tolerated, but adequate loop distension strictly depends on patient compliance, because patients are asked to drink a large volume of liquids (eg, 1000–2000 mL) in a short time frame (approximately 1.5–2 h), according to a predefined schedule, which varies across centers. The choice between the 2 approaches remains controversial and depends on several factors, such as expected disease location, local radiology practice, and the diagnostic algorithms of different centers. Nevertheless, enterography is frequently used in everyday clinical practice, given its better patient tolerance and acceptability.[67–71]

In conjunction with luminal contrast agents, intravenous iodinated contrast agents are also administered to optimize the assessment of small bowel during CT; although gadolinium-based contrast agents are not always required during MR studies, they are generally used when assessing inflammatory or potentially malignant small bowel processes (**Fig. 6**). Antispasmodic agents (ie, hyoscine butylbromide or glucagon) are also routinely administered intravenously at time of examination to reduce artifact due to peristaltic contractions.

MRI has been shown more sensitive than CT for detecting mucosal lesions of the small bowel, and it seems to facilitate the identification of subtle mucosal changes.[71] These

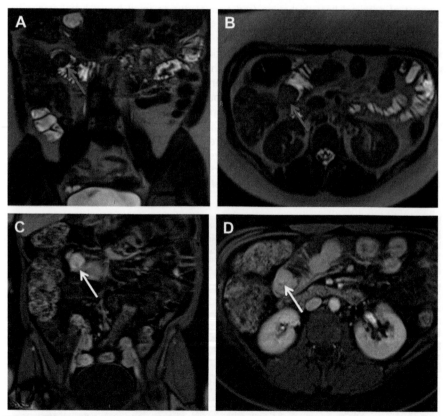

Fig. 6. Jejunal small bowel GISTs. MR enterography: coronal (*A*) and axial (*B*) views of jejunal GIST (marked by the *red arrows* in panels *A* and *B*). Postgadolinium MRIs (coronal [*C*] and axial [*D*]) views demonstrate enhancement of the jejunal GIST (marked by the *red arrows* in panels *C* and *D*).

findings may be due to the better soft tissue contrast that can be achieved with MRI; diffusion-weighted imaging is now a standard sequence while performing MR small bowel imaging because it improves the detection of small bowel tumors and inflammatory small bowel pathology.[72–74] Recent data seem to suggest that for the specific subset of small bowel tumors, MR has higher diagnostic performance compared with CT.[75] Moreover, because of the exposure to ionizing radiation with CT, the latter can be performed at only a few time points.[68] Therefore, repeated dynamic imaging, and hence assessment of small bowel peristaltic activity, is not usually possible with CT, and an intermittent spasm or peristaltic contraction during the CT examination can also be misdiagnosed as a small bowel neoplasm.[76] Nevertheless, the use of the latest generation of multidetector CT scanners and specific acquisition protocols can significantly reduce the radiation dose.[77,78] It has also been shown that CT produced higher-quality images, mostly due to rapid acquisition, compared with MR[75] and it seems to have better performance than MR in the assessment of potential perforation or complete bowel obstruction.[65] CT is more frequently performed in patients who have difficulty in holding their breath or in those presenting with acute abdomen, whereas MR is preferred in young patients or in those with known renal impairment, in whom the administration of intravenous iodinated contrast agent can worsen renal function. In everyday clinical practice, however, MRI is less readily available and more time consuming.[67,68] Taking into account the pros and cons of CT and MR techniques in the setting of suspected small bowel tumors, the choice between them often relies on opportunistic reasons (availability, local expertise, costs, and radiologist preference), rather than on clinical or technical issues.

The use of dedicated small bowel cross-sectional imaging techniques allows accurate detection of small bowel tumors with sensitivities and specificities of 85 to 94 and 95% to 97%, respectively.[67,68,79] Furthermore, some studies report excellent interobserver agreement.[67,80] Although the overall sensitivity of radiologic imaging tests can be influenced by the small number of patients included in single studies and by strict patient selection (in a majority of studies, only patients with suspected small bowel tumors were included), both CT and MR seem excellent diagnostic techniques for detecting small bowel tumors. As for CE, however, both CT and MR radiologic imaging techniques lack specificity to differentiate between different subtypes of tumors. Although different small bowel tumors have characteristic imaging features,[81,82] no feature is absolutely specific. The identification of small bowel tumors by radiologic imaging warrants further examinations, aimed at obtaining tissue samples.

Cases of false-positive (ie, patients with adhesions or inflammatory bowel thickening) and false-negative examinations (in which the final diagnosis has been reached by other techniques) have been reported. Despite the highlighted limitations, however, dedicated small bowel cross-sectional imaging techniques have an obvious advantage over endoscopic tests for the study of the small bowel: they allow detailed panoramic extraluminal evaluation, providing diagnosis and staging at the same time. For this reason, when they are not used as first-line examination (eg, in patients with occlusion), radiologic examinations are almost universally performed in the diagnostic work-up of small bowel tumors, as a confirmatory or preoperative test.

There are other advanced radiologic techniques (ie, octreoscan and PET with gallium 68), not discussed in this article, which are essential diagnostic tests as far as specific tumors (ie, neuroendocrine) of the small bowel are suspected.

DEVICE-ASSISTED ENTEROSCOPY

The rate of small bowel tumors diagnosed in patients undergoing DAE for mixed clinical indications is approximately 10% (**Table 1**).[32,83–96] Nevertheless, there is

Table 1
Rate of small bowel tumors diagnosed in large cohorts of patients (≥100) undergoing device-assisted enteroscopy for mixed indications

Author, Ref Year	Patients Undergoing Device-assisted Enteroscopy	Patients with Small Bowl Tumor (%)	Study Time Frame	Country
Zhong et al,[83] 2007	378	63 (16.7)	2003–2005	China
Li et al,[84] 2007	218	7 (3.2)	NR	China
Mitsui et al,[85] 2009	1035	144 (13.9)	2005–2010	Japan
Lee et al,[86] 2011	645	112 (17.4)	2004–2009	Korea
Imaoka et al,[87] 2011	227	20 (8.8)	2005–2010	Japan
Honda et al,[32] 2012	806	159 (19.7)	2003–2011	Japan
Eastern countries (cumulative)	*3309*	*505 (15.2)*	*NA*	*NA*
Heine et al,[88] 2006	275	15 (5.4)	2003–2005	Netherlands
Cazzato et al,[89] 2007	100	7 (7.0)	2004–2006	Italy
Hegde et al,[90] 2010	176	23 (13.0)	2007–2008	United States
Morgan et al,[91] 2010	148	10 (6.8)	2008	United States
Partridge et al,[92] 2011	555	20 (3.6)	2004–2009	United States
Manno et al,[93] 2013	111	15 (13.5)	2010–2011	Italy
Cangemi et al,[94] 2013	1106	134 (12.1)	2005–2012	United States
Pérez-Cuadrado et al,[95] 2015	627	28 (4.5)	2004–2014	Spain
Pinho et al,[96] 2016	1411	71 (5.0)	2003–2013	Portugal
Western countries (cumulative)	*4509*	*323 (7.1)*	*NA*	*NA*
Overall	7818	828 (10.6)	NA	NA

wide variability amongst studies (range 3%–20%). The variability depends on several factors. First, the articles from Eastern countries report a higher rate of small bowel tumors (approximately und 15%), as also observed in CE studies.[51] This likely reflects different patient selection (eg, in the study from Mitsui and colleagues,[85] the rate of small bowel tumors dropped from 13.9% to 7.3% when Peutz-Jeghers patients were excluded) as well as the different utilization of DAE in different countries. Second, in some series, both benign and malignant tumors were included; and last, in some of them, only histologically confirmed tumors were taken into account.

As far as the accuracy of DAE in diagnosing small bowel tumors or polyps is concerned, a recent meta-analysis[97] of 15 studies and 821 patients reported that sensitivity, specificity, and positive and negative predictive value were 89%, 97%, 16.6, and 0.14, respectively. DAE is often performed, however, when another diagnostic technique has already shown the presence of a possible small bowel tumor. Thus, the contribution of DAE mostly relies on a couple of features, crucial for planning further management, that is, ability for tissue sampling and a more precise localization of the lesion. As previously shown, CE lacks specificity. Similarly, although some tumors have specific CT or MRI features, in a majority of cases a definite histologic diagnosis is impossible with these techniques. DAE can help in bridging this gap.

The effectiveness of enteroscopy biopsies in reaching a histologic diagnosis is high, although variable across studies (range 70%–100%) (**Table 2**).[32,86,87,95] In addition, a consistent agreement between histologic and laparoscopic resected specimens has been shown.[98] Nevertheless, in up to 30% of cases, although an obvious mucosal lesion is reached, biopsies are negative. On one hand, this could be due to technical difficulties in performing adequate biopsies (ie, small working channel of some scopes or unstable scope position in the distal small bowel). On the other hand, in 80% of cases in which DAE biopsies missed the diagnosis, the lesions were of subepithelial origin[32,87,94,97] (**Fig. 7**). Additionally, some investigators[32] raised concerns about taking several biopsies from small bowel subepithelial tumors, because they are prone to massive bleeding.

Even when a definite histologic diagnosis is not reachable, DAE allows localization of the lesion, by measuring the distance from reliable anatomic landmarks, and more importantly, by marking the identified lesion (by means of India ink (**Fig. 8**), Lipiodol, or clip placement). Marking a small bowel tumour represents a critical step in the management of small bowel tumors, because the introduction of minimally invasive surgical procedures makes the palpatory exploration of the entire organ unfeasible. Nowadays, in the setting of small bowel tumors, the combination of DAE and laparoscopy represents an ideal therapeutic method.[98]

In a recent multicenter Korean study,[86] the investigators reported that therapeutic plans had been changed after DAE in more than 60% of patients with small bowel tumors. Pérez-Cuadrado and colleagues[95] detailed the change in management due to DAE results, including delaying or avoiding emergency surgery, modifying surgery approach, and indicating small bowel partial resection, instead of elective approach.

Unfortunately, DAE techniques have some inherent limitations: the procedure is time consuming and requires a trained team and deep sedation. In addition, total enteroscopy cannot be performed in all patients and therapeutic interventions, including hemostasis, polypectomy, and stenting, are associated with an adverse event rate up to 10% (mostly polipectomy related), including perforation, pancreatitis, and bleeding.[99,100]

To overcome the limitations of currently available device-assisted enteroscopes, new prototypes with a wider (3.2-mm) operative channel or lower outer diameter, as well as automated spiral enteroscopes, which would enable an extremely easy, quick, and complete small bowel evaluation requiring only 1 trained endoscopist instead of a large team, are under evaluation.

SMALL BOWEL TUMORS DIAGNOSTIC WORK-UP: FROM EVIDENCE TO CLINICAL PRACTICE

Given the results of clinical studies and limitations of the individual diagnostic tools, the available evidence highlights that the diagnostic tests described in this review

Table 2
Effectiveness of device-assisted enteroscopy histologic confirmation of small bowel tumors across studies

Author, Ref Year	Histologic Diagnosis
Lee et al,[86] 2011	72.9%
Imaoka et al,[87] 2011	100.0%
Honda et al,[32] 2012	90.1%
Pérez-Cuadrado et al,[95] 2015	71.4%

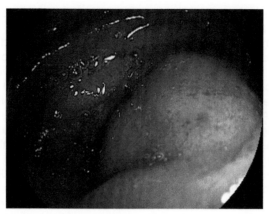

Fig. 7. Small bowel GIST identified by DAE.

are, in the setting of patients with small bowel tumors, absolutely complementary, rather than alternative. In this setting, the result of a single test is often insufficient for establishing a definite diagnosis or ruling out the presence of small bowel tumor. Conversely, a reasoned and balanced combination of the different tests allows to overcome the limitations of each single procedure to reach a final diagnosis or to decrease the level of uncertainty.

A possible algorithmic approach for the evaluation of patients with suspected small bowel tumor is presented in **Fig. 9**. Although this is based on available clinical evidence and pros/cons of single diagnostic tools, the diagnostic work-up for individual patients in everyday clinical practice heavily depends on local expertise and availability of different techniques as well as on organizational and economic issues. These instances can explain geographic and procedural differences observed in different studies.

When a small bowel tumor is suspected, the diagnostic work-up ideally should start with the least invasive and the panoramic diagnostic tools (namely, CE or dedicated cross-sectional radiologic imaging) depending on patient characteristics and clinical presentation.

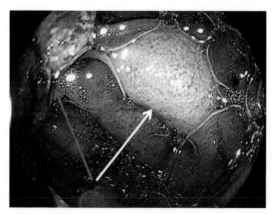

Fig. 8. Actively bleeding small bowel cavernous hemangioma (*red arrow*) with tattoo (*white arrow*).

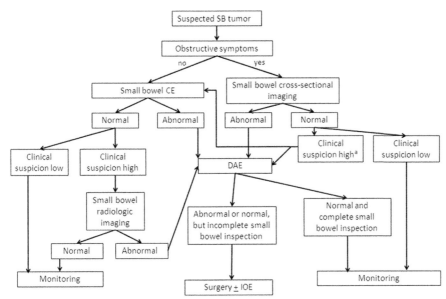

Fig. 9. Algorithmic approach for the evaluation of patient with suspected small bowel tumor. [a] In patients with obstructive symptoms when the clinical suspicion remains high, despite negative cross-sectional imaging, further small bowel investigations should be considered; in this case, the choice between DAE and small bowel CE should be done on a case-by-case basis. [b] In patients without obstructive symptoms, when CE is positive and DAE is normal but incomplete, dedicated small bowel cross-sectional imaging should be considered before surgery. IOE, intraoperative enteroscopy; SB, small bowel.

When a small bowel tumor is suspected and there are no obstructive features, CE should be considered the ideal first-line investigation, mostly because small bowel tumors may present with obscure GI bleeding in several cases. If CE is positive, a further examination aimed at reaching a final histologic diagnosis (namely DAE) is warranted. Where DAE is guided by a previous positive CE, especially when a small bowel tumor is suspected, its diagnostic yield significantly increases.[101,102] In this setting, CE can also indicate the most efficient DAE approach (per oral or per anal). When the lesion, identified by CE, is close to the pylorus or the ileocecal valve, push enteroscopy instead of DAE can be successfully performed.[103] Furthermore, if a lesion is located within the first 60% to 75%[104,105] of the capsule small bowel transit time, DAE through the oral approach has a higher chance of reaching the targeted lesion, precisely locating it, and finally reaching the final diagnosis by taking tissue samples. Last but not least, DAE may allow retrieval of retained capsules.[106] Even economic models highlight that a diagnostic strategy in which the capsule is performed as first test results in cost savings.[107] Nevertheless, as discussed previously, CE can miss small bowel tumors, which can be successfully identified by either DAE or dedicated small bowel cross-sectional radiologic imaging.[43,108] Because the latter is less invasive, readily available, and provides a complete evaluation of the entire small bowel in a single examination, it takes precedence over DAE. Whenever initial CE and subsequent dedicated small bowel cross-sectional imaging tests are both negative, clinical re-evaluation of patients and individualized watchful monitoring seem reasonable.

Dedicated small bowel cross-sectional imaging techniques can also represent the first-line test, when CE is unavailable or contraindicated, as in patients with obstruction. In some series, including several patients with small bowel tumors, dedicated cross-sectional radiologic tests show performance characteristics similar or superior to those of endoscopic methods.[44–110] When small bowel dedicated cross-sectional radiologic tests, used as first diagnostic test, result as positive, they can be confirmed by DAE or directly by surgical intervention, if DAE is contraindicated or unavailable or when the complete small bowel exploration fails. Even small bowel dedicated cross-sectional radiologic tests can effectively drive the selection of the insertion route, and histologic diagnosis, reached by means of DAE, allows planning of further diagnostic/therapeutic maneuvers. Again, taking into account limitation of small bowel dedicated cross-sectional radiologic tests, when the initial examination is negative, but clinical suspicion remains high, endoscopic methods should be considered. It is extremely important, however, to emphasize that the definition of "clinical suspicion of small intestinal tumor" is far from standardized.

ACKNOWLEDGMENTS

We sincerely thank Stephen Glancy (Department of Radiology, Western General Hospital, Edinburgh, Scotland) and Panagiota Demosthenous (Department of Electrical and Computer Engineering, University of Cyprus, Cyprus) for their contributions to this article.

REFERENCES

1. Neugut AI, Jacobson JS, Suh S, et al. The epidemiology of cancer of the small bowel. Cancer Epidemiol Biomarkers Prev 1998;7:243–51.
2. Rossini FP, Risio M, Pennazio M. Small bowel tumors and polyposis syndromes. Gastrointest Endosc Clin N Am 1999;9:93–114.
3. Di Sario JA, Burt RW, Vargas H, et al. Small bowel cancer: epidemiological and clinical characteristics from a population-based registry. Am J Gastroenterol 1994;89:699–701.
4. O'Riordan BG, Vilor M, Herrera L. Small bowel tumors: an overview. Dig Dis Sci 1996;14:245–57.
5. Pan SY, Morrison H. Epidemiology of cancer oft he small intestine. World J Gastroint Onc 2011;3:33–42.
6. Islam RS, Leighton JA, Pasha SF. Evaluation and management of small-bowel tumors in the era of deep enteroscopy. Gastrointest Endosc 2014;79:732–40.
7. National Cancer Institute. SEER stat fact sheets: small intestine cancer. Available at: http://seer.cancer.gov/statfacts/html/smint.html. Accessed 25 March, 2016.
8. Ross RK, Hartnett NM, Bernstein L, et al. Epidemiology of adenocarcinomas of the small intestine: is bile a small bowel carcinogen? Br J Cancer 1991;63: 143–5.
9. Weiss NS, Yang CP. Incidence of histologic types of cancer of the small intestine. J Natl Cancer Inst 1987;78:653–6.
10. Gabos S, Berkel J, Band P, et al. Small bowel cancer in western Canada. Int J Epidemiol 1993;22:198–206.
11. Chow JS, Chen CC, Ahsan H, et al. A population-based study of the incidence of malignant small bowel tumours: SEER, 1973-1990. Int J Epidemiol 1996;25: 722–8.

12. Severson RK, Schenk M, Gurney JG, et al. Increasing incidence of adenocarcinomas and carcinoid tumors of the small intestine in adults. Cancer Epidemiol Biomarkers Prev 1996;5:81–4.
13. Hatzaras I, Palesty JA, Abir F, et al. Small-bowel tumors: epidemiologic and clinical characteristics of 1260 cases from the Connecticut tumor registry. Arch Surg 2007;142:229–35.
14. Blanchard DK, Budde JM, Hatch GF 3rd, et al. Tumors of the Small Intestine. World J Surg 2000;24:421–9.
15. Haselkorn T, Whittemore AS, Lilienfeld DE. Incidence of small bowel cancer in the United States and worldwide: geographic, temporal, and racial differences. Cancer Causes Control 2005;16:781–7.
16. Shack LG, Wood HE, Kang JY, et al. Small intestinal cancer in England & Wales and Scotland: time trends in incidence, mortality and survival. Aliment Pharmacol Ther 2006;23:1297–306.
17. Lu Y, Fröbom R, Lagergren J. Incidence patterns of small bowel cancer in a population-based study in Sweden: increase in duodenal adenocarcinoma. Cancer Epidemiol 2012;36:e158–63.
18. Lepage C, Bouvier AM, Manfredi S, et al. Incidence and management of primary malignant small bowel cancers: a well-defined French population study. Am J Gastroenterol 2006;101:2826–32.
19. Bojesen RD, Andersson M, Riis LB, et al. Incidence of, phenotypes of and survival from small bowel cancer in Denmark, 1994-2010: a population-based study. J Gastroenterol 2016;51(9):891–9.
20. Wolk A, Gridley G, Svensson M, et al. A prospective study of obesity and cancer risk (Sweden). Cancer Causes Control 2001;12:13–21.
21. Samanic C, Gridley G, Chow WH, et al. Obesity and cancer risk among white and black United States veterans. Cancer Causes Control 2004;15:35–43.
22. Chen CC, Neugut AI, Rotterdam H. Risk factors for adenocarcinomas and malignant carcinoids of the small intestine: preliminary findings. Cancer Epidemiol Biomarkers Prev 1994;3:205–7.
23. Wu AH, Yu MC, Mack TM. Smoking, alcohol use, dietary factors and risk of small intestinal adenocarcinoma. Int J Cancer 1997;70:512–7.
24. Kaerlev L, Teglbjaerg PS, Sabroe S, et al. The importance of smoking and medical history for development of small bowel carcinoid tumor: a European population-based case-control study. Cancer Causes Control 2002;13: 27–34.
25. Hamilton SR, Aaltonen LA. World health organization classification of tumours. Pathology and genetics of tumours of the digestive system. Chapter 4. Lyon (France): IARC Press; 2000. p. 69–92.
26. Wu TJ, Yeh CN, Chao TC, et al. Prognostic factors of primary small bowel adenocarcinoma: univariate and multivariate analysis. World J Surg 2006;30: 391–8.
27. Talamonti MS, Goetz LH, Rao S, et al. Primary cancers of the small bowel: analysis of prognostic factors and results of surgical management. Arch Surg 2002; 137:564–70 [discussion: 570–1].
28. George S, Trent JC. The role of imatinib plasma level testing in gastrointestinal stromal tumor. Cancer Chemother Pharmacol 2011;67(Suppl 1):S45–50.
29. Essat M, Cooper K. Imatinib as adjuvant therapy for gastrointestinal stromal tumors: a systematic review. Int J Cancer 2011;128:2202–14.
30. Kala Z, Válek V, Kysela P, et al. A shift in the diagnostics of the small intestine tumors. Eur J Radiol 2007;62:160–5.

31. Cardoso H, Rodrigues J, Marques M, et al. Malignant small bowel tumors: diagnosis, management and prognosis. Acta Med Port 2015;28:448–56.

32. Honda W, Ohmiya N, Hirooka Y, et al. Enteroscopic and radiologic diagnoses, treatment, and prognoses of small-bowel tumors. Gastrointest Endosc 2012; 76:344–54.

33. Anderson LA, Tavilla A, Brenner H, et al. Survival for oesophageal, stomach and small intestine cancers in Europe 1999-2007: results from EUROCARE-5. Eur J Cancer 2015;51:2144–57.

34. Cobrin GM, Pittman RH, Lewis BS. Increased diagnostic yield of small bowel tumors with capsule endoscopy. Cancer 2006;107:22–7.

35. Urbain D, De Looze D, Demedts I, et al. Video capsule endoscopy in small-bowel malignancy: a multicenter Belgian study. Endoscopy 2006;38:408–11.

36. Pasha SF, Sharma VK, Carey EJ, et al. A single center experience of 1000 consecutive patients. Proceedings of the 6th International Conference on Capsule Endoscopy. Madrid (Spain), June 8–10, 2007. p. 45.

37. Rondonotti E, Pennazio M, Toth E, et al. Small-bowel neoplasms in patients undergoing video capsule endoscopy: a multicenter European study. Endoscopy 2008;40:488–95.

38. Lim YJ, Lee OY, Jeen YT, et al. Indication for detection, completion and retention rates of small bowel capsule endoscopy based on the 10-years data from the Korean Capsule Endoscopy Registry. Clin Endosc 2015;48:399–404.

39. Cheung DY, Lee IS, Chang DK, et al. Capsule endoscopy in small bowel tumors: a multicenter Korean Study. J Gastroenterol Hepatol 2010;25:1079–86.

40. Koulaouzidis A, Yung DE, Lam JHP, et al. The use of small-bowel capsule endoscopy in iron-deficiency anemia alone; be aware of the young anemic patient. Scand J Gastroenterol 2012;47:1094–100.

41. Sidhu R, McAlindon ME, Drew K, et al. Evaluating the role of small-bowel endoscopy in clinical practice: the largest single-centre experience. Eur J Gastroenterol Hepatol 2012;24:513–9.

42. Lewis BS, Eisen GM, Friedman S. A pooled analysis to evaluate results of capsule endoscopy trials. Endoscopy 2005;37:960–5.

43. Ross A, Mehdizadeh S, Tokar J, et al. Double balloon enteroscopy detects small bowel mass lesions missed by capsule endoscopy. Dig Dis Sci 2008;53:2140–3.

44. Huprich JE, Fletcher JG, Fidler JL, et al. Prospective blinded comparison of wireless capsule endoscopy and multiphase CT enterography in obscure gastrointestinal bleeding. Radiology 2011;260:744–51.

45. Klein A, Dashkovsky M, Gralnek I, et al. Bowel preparation in "real-life" small bowel capsule endoscopy: a two-center experience. Ann Gastroenterol 2016; 29:196–200.

46. Worsoe J, Fynne L, Gregersen T, et al. Gastric transit and small intestinal transit time and motility assessed by amagnet tracking system. BMC Gastroenterol 2011;11:145.

47. Appleyard M, Fireman Z, Glukhovsky A, et al. A randomized trial comparing wireless capsule endoscopy with push enteroscopy for the detection of small-bowel lesions. Gastroenterology 2000;119:1431–8.

48. Koulaouzidis A, Rondonotti E, Karargyris A. Small-bowel capsule endoscopy: A ten-point contemporary. World J Gastroenterol 2013;19:3726–46.

49. Friedrich K, Gehrke S, Stremmel W, et al. First clinical trial of a newly developed capsule endoscope with panoramic side view for small bowel: a pilot study. J Gastroenterol Hepatol 2013;28:1496–501.

50. Esaki M, Matsumoto T, Kudo T, et al. Bowel preparations for capsule endoscopy: a comparison between simethicone and magnesium citrate. Gastrointest Endosc 2009;69(1):94–101.
51. Liao Z, Gao R, Xu C, et al. Indications and detection, completion, and retention rates of small-bowel capsule endoscopy: a systematic review. Gastrointest Endosc 2010;71:280–6.
52. Song HJ, Moon JS, Shim KN. Optimal Bowel Preparation for Video Capsule Endoscopy. Gastroenterol Res Pract 2016;2016:6802810.
53. Song HJ, Moon JS, Do JH, et al. Guidelines for Bowel Preparation before Video Capsule Endoscopy. Clin Endosc 2013;46:147–54.
54. Mathus-Vliegen E, Pellisé M, Heresbach D, et al. Consensus guidelines for the use of bowel preparation prior to colonic diagnostic procedures: colonoscopy and small bowel video capsule endoscopy. Curr Med Res Opin 2013;29: 931–45.
55. Shiotani A, Honda K, Kawakami M, et al. Use of an external real-time image viewer coupled with prespecified actions enhanced the complete examinations for capsule endoscopy. J Gastroenterol Hepatol 2011;26:1270–4.
56. Girelli CM, Porta P, Colombo E, et al. Development of a novel index to discriminate bulge from mass on small-bowel capsule endoscopy. Gastrointest Endosc 2011;74:1067–74.
57. Shyung LR, Lin SC, Shih SC, et al. Proposed scoring system to determine small bowel mass lesions using capsule endoscopy. J Formos Med Assoc 2009;108: 533–8.
58. Rondonotti E, Koulaouzidis A, Karargyris A, et al. Utility of 3-dimensional image reconstruction in the diagnosis of small-bowel masses in capsule endoscopy (with video). Gastrointest Endosc 2014;80:642–51.
59. Pennazio M, Spada C, Eliakim R, et al. Small-bowel capsule endoscopy and device-assisted enteroscopy for diagnosis and treatment of small-bowel disorders: European Society of Gastrointestinal Endoscopy (ESGE) Clinical Guideline. Endoscopy 2015;47:352–76.
60. Van Gossum A. Image-enhanced capsule endoscopy for characterization of small bowel lesions. Best Pract Res Clin Gastroenterol 2015;29:525–31.
61. Ryu CB, Song JY, Lee MS, et al. Mo1670 Does Capsule Endoscopy With Alice Improves Visibility of Small Bowel Lesions? Gastrointest Endosc 2013;77: AB466.
62. Demosthenous P, Pitris C, Georgiou J. Infrared Fluorescence-Based Cancer Screening Capsule for the Small Intestine. IEEE Trans Biomed Circuits Syst 2016;10:467–76.
63. Akbari H, Halig LV, Zhang H, et al. Detection of cancer metastasis using a novel macroscopic hyperspectral method. Proc SPIE Int Soc Opt Eng 2012;8317: 831711.
64. Lu G, Halig L, Wang D, et al. Hyperspectral imaging for cancer surgical margin delineation: registration of hyperspectral and histological images. Proc SPIE Int Soc Opt Eng 2014;90360S:90360S.
65. Zamboni GA, Raptopoulos V. CT enterography. Gastrointest Endosc Clin N Am 2010;20:347–66.
66. Schmidt SA, Baumann JA, Stanescu-Siegmund N, et al. Oral distension methods for small bowel MRI: comparison of different agents to optimize bowel distension. Acta Radiol 2016. [Epub ahead of print].
67. Faggian A, Fracella MR, D'Alesio G, et al. Small-Bowel Neoplasms: Role of MRI Enteroclysis. Gastroenterol Res Pract 2016;2016:9686815.

68. Masselli G, Gualdi G. CT and MR enterography in evaluating small bowel diseases: when to use which modality? Abdom Imaging 2013;38:249–59.
69. Arrivé L, El Mouhadi S. MR enterography versus MR enteroclysis. Radiology 2013;266:688.
70. Kishi T, Shimizu K, Hashimoto S, et al. CT enteroclysis/enterography findings in drug-induced small-bowel damage. Br J Radiol 2014;87:20140367.
71. Horsthuis K, Stokkers PC, Stoker J. Detection of inflammatory bowel disease: diagnostic performance of cross-sectional imaging modalities. Abdom Imaging 2011;33:407–16.
72. Amzallag-Bellenger E, Soyer P, Barbe C, et al. Diffusion-weighted imaging for the detection of mesenteric small bowel tumours with Magnetic Resonance–enterography. Eur Radiol 2014;24:2916–26.
73. Sinha R, Rajiah P, Ramachandran I, et al. Diffusion-weighted MR imaging of the gastrointestinal tract: technique, indications, and imaging findings. Radiographics 2013;33:655–76.
74. Fidler JL, Guimaraes L, Einstein DM. MR imaging of the small bowel. Radiographics 2009;29:1811–25.
75. Masselli G, Di Tola M, Casciani E, et al. Diagnosis of Small-Bowel Diseases: Prospective Comparison of Multi-Detector Row CT Enterography with MR Enterography. Radiology 2016;279:420–31.
76. Maglinte DD, Sandrasegaran K, Lappas JC, et al. CT enteroclysis. Radiology 2007;245:661–71.
77. Fletcher JG, Fidler JL, Bruining DH, et al. New concepts in intestinal imaging for inflammatory bowel diseases. Gastroenterology 2011;140:1795–806.
78. Siddiki HA, Fidler JL, Fletcher JG, et al. Prospective comparison of state-of-the-art MR enterography and CT-enterography in small bowel Crohn's disease. Am J Roentgenol 2009;193:113–21.
79. Soyer P, Aout M, Hoeffel C, et al. Helical CT-enteroclysis in the detection of small-bowel tumours: a meta-analysis. Eur Radiol 2013;23:388–99.
80. Booya F, Fletcher JG, Huprich JE, et al. Active Crohn disease: CT findings and interobserver agreement for enteric phase CT enterography. Radiology 2006; 241:787–95.
81. Sailer J, Zacherl J, Schima W. MDCT of small bowel tumours. Cancer Imaging 2007;7:224–33.
82. Anzidei M, Napoli A, Zini C, et al. Malignant tumours of the small intestine: a review of histopathology, multidetector CT and MRI aspects. Br J Radiol 2011;84: 677–90.
83. Zhong J, Ma T, Zhang C, et al. A retrospective study of the application on double-balloon enteroscopy in 378 patients with suspected small bowel diseases. Endoscopy 2007;39:208–15.
84. Li XB, Ge ZZ, Dai J, et al. The role of capsule endoscopy combined with double-balloon enteroscopy in diagnosis of small bowel diseases. Chin Med J 2007; 120:30–5.
85. Mitsui K, Tanaka S, Yamamoto H, et al. Role of double-balloon endoscopy in the diagnosis of small bowel tumors: the first Japanese multicenter study. Gastrointest Endosc 2009;70:498–504.
86. Lee BL, Choi H, Choi KY, et al. Clinical characteristics of small bowel tumors diagnosed by double-balloon endoscopy: KASID multi-center study. Dig Dis Sci 2011;56:2920–7.
87. Imaoka H, Higaki N, Kumagi T, et al. Characteristics of small bowel tumors detected by double balloon endoscopy. Dig Dis Sci 2011;56:2366–71.

88. Heine GD, Hadithi M, Groenen MJM, et al. Double-balloon enteroscopy: indications, diagnostic yield and complications in a series of 275 patients with suspected small bowel disease. Endoscopy 2006;38:42–8.

89. Cazzato IA, Cammarota G, Nista EC, et al. Diagnostic and therapeutic impact of double-baloon enteroscopy in a series of 100 patients with suspected small bowel lesions. Dig Liv Dis 2007;39:483–7.

90. Hegde SR, Iffrig K, Li T, et al. double balloon enteroscopy in the elderly: safety, findings, and diagnostic and therapeutic success. Gastrointest Endosc 2010; 71:983–9.

91. Morgan D, Upchurch B, Draganov P, et al. Spiral enteroscopy: prospective U.S. multicenter study in patients with small-bowel disorders. Gastrointest Endosc 2010;72:992–8.

92. Partridge BJ, Tokar JL, Haluszka O, et al. Small bowel cancers diagnosed by device-assisted enteroscopy at a U.S. referral centre: a five-year experience. Dig Dis Sci 2011;56:2701–5.

93. Manno M, Riccioni ME, Cannizzaro R, et al. Diagnostic and therapeutic yield of single balloon enteroscopy inpatients with suspected small-bowel disease: results of the Italian multicenter study. Dig Liv Dis 2013;45:211–5.

94. Cangemi DJ, Patel MK, Gomez V, et al. Small bowel tumors discovered during double-balloon enteroscopy. Analysis of a large prospectively collected single-center database. J Clin Gastroenterol 2013;47:769–72.

95. Pérez-Cuadrado E, Delgado PE, Conesa PB, et al. Role of double-balloon enteroscopy in malignant small bowel tumors. World J Gastrointest Endosc 2015;7:652–8.

96. Pinho R, Mascarenhas-Saraiva M, Mao-de-Ferro S, et al. Multicenter survey on the use of device-assisted enteroscopy in Portugal. United Eur Gastroenterol J 2016;4:264–74.

97. Sulbaran M, de Moura E, Bernardo W, et al. Overtube-assisted enteroscopy and capsule endoscopy for the diagnosis of small-bowel polyps and tumors: a systematic review and meta-analysis. Endosc Int Open 2016;04:E151–63.

98. Riccioni ME, Cianci R, Urgesi R, et al. Advance in diagnosis and treatment of small bowel tumors: a single-center report. Surg Endosc 2012;26:438–41.

99. Chavalitdhamrong D, Adler DG, Draganov PV. Complications of enteroscopy: how to avoid them and manage them when they arise. Gastrointest Endosc Clin N Am 2015;25:83–95.

100. Moeschler O, Mueller MK. Deep enteroscopy-indications, diagnostic yield and complications. World J Gastroenterol 2015;21:1385–93.

101. Sethi S, Cohen J, Thaker AM, et al. Prior capsule endoscopy improves the diagnostic and therapeutic yield of single-balloon enteroscopy. Dig Dis Sci 2014;59: 2497–502.

102. Teshima CW, Kuipers EJ, van Zanten SV, et al. Double balloon enteroscopy and capsule endoscopy for obscure gastrointestinal bleeding: an updated meta-analysis. J Gastroenterol Hepatol 2011;26:796–801.

103. Modi C, Desai AD, De Pasquale JR, et al. Push enteroscopy: a useful modality for proximal small-bowel mass lesions. J Gastrointest Canc 2013;44: 347–50.

104. Li X, Chen H, Dai J, et al. Predictive role of capsule endoscopy on the insertion route of double-balloon enteroscopy. Endoscopy 2009;41:762–6.

105. Gay G, Delvaux M, Fassler I. Outcome of capsule endoscopy in determining indication and route for push-and-pull enteroscopy. Endoscopy 2006;38:49–58.

106. Van Weyenberg SJ, Van Turenhout ST, Bouma G, et al. Double-balloon endoscopy as the primary method forsmall-bowel video capsule endoscope retrieval. Gastrointest Endosc 2010;71:535–41.
107. Albert JG, Nachtigall F, Wiedbrauck F, et al. Minimizing procedural cost in diagnosing small bowel bleeding: comparison of a strategy based on initial capsule endoscopy versus initial double-balloon enteroscopy. Eur J Gastroenterol Hepatol 2010;22:679–88.
108. Postgate A, Despott E, Burling D, et al. Significant small-bowel lesions detected by alternative diagnostic modalities after negative capsule endoscopy. Gastrointest Endosc 2008;68:1209–14.
109. Wang J, Guo Q, Zhao J, et al. Multidetector ct enterography versus double-balloon enteroscopy: comparison of the diagnostic value for patients with suspected small bowel diseases. Gastroenterol Res Pract 2016;2016:5172873.
110. Khalife S, Soyer P, Alatawi A, et al. Obscure gastrointestinal bleeding: preliminary comparison of 64-section CT enteroclysis with video capsule endoscopy. Eur Radiol 2011;21:79–86.

Double-Balloon Enteroscopy

Andrea May, MD

KEYWORDS

- Double-balloon enteroscopy (DBE) • Balloon-assisted enteroscopy
- Midgastrointestinal bleeding (MGIB) • Complete enteroscopy • Diagnostic DBE
- Therapeutic DBE

KEY POINTS

- Double-balloon enteroscopy (DBE) was the first flexible technique for achieving deep small bowel endoscopy without the need for surgery.
- Proper patient selection and device selection are mandatory for successful diagnosis and treatment.
- Skill in enteroscopy and in the management of small bowel diseases is the key to successful enteroscopy.
- DBE provides the highest rate of complete enteroscopy if complete enteroscopy is needed.
- Obscure bleeding should no longer be used as a synonym for small bowel bleeding, but should be limited to gastrointestinal bleeding of unclear origin after a negative diagnostic work-up including enteroscopy.

INTRODUCTION

Since the introduction of double-balloon enteroscopy (DBE) 15 years ago, flexible enteroscopy has become an established method in the diagnostic and therapeutic work-up of small bowel disorders. Various techniques for deep small bowel endoscopy have been developed since then, and are described in detail in other articles in this issue. All of the methods can be summed up under the generic term device-assisted enteroscopy. There are 2 main subgroups. First, there are balloon enteroscopy techniques, which all follow the push-and-pull principle; by contrast, spiral enteroscopy is based on the principle of rotation.[1–4] Balloon enteroscopy can be further subdivided into 2 groups: balloon-guided enteroscopy and balloon-assisted enteroscopy, which can be performed with either 1 balloon (single-balloon enteroscopy [SBE]) or 2 balloons (DBE). **Fig. 1** provides an overview of the different techniques. DBE was the first method introduced that allowed flexible enteroscopy

Department of Gastroenterology, Sana Klinikum Offenbach GmbH, Starkenburgring 66, Offenbach am Main 63069, Germany
E-mail address: andrea.may@sana.de

Gastrointest Endoscopy Clin N Am 27 (2017) 113–122
http://dx.doi.org/10.1016/J.glec.2016.08.006
1052-5157/17/© 2016 Elsevier Inc. All rights reserved.

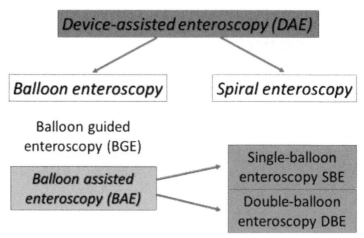

Fig. 1. Overview of the different techniques for deep small bowel endoscopy.

without the need for surgery, and it is therefore also now the oldest.[5–10] Considerable experience has been gained with the method in recent years, and most studies and publications on enteroscopy have been performed using DBE (**Fig. 2**). This article provides an update on the indications for DBE, performance of the technique, and outcomes associated with it.

Indications

Any type of known or suspected small bowel disease may be an indication for an examination of the small bowel for either diagnostic or therapeutic purposes. Flexible small bowel endoscopy is generally performed for diagnosis, to check unclear lesions that have been identified using other imaging techniques, such as capsule or radiological methods; to obtain histologic data through biopsy sampling; or in patients with continuing symptoms and previously negative diagnostic work-up in whom there is

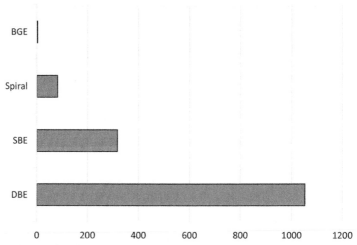

Fig. 2. Numbers of publications associated with the different types of enteroscopy, including original publications, reviews, case series, and case reports, listed in PubMed.

a suspicion of a small bowel disorder. Therapeutic interventions include marking the bowel wall with India ink before laparoscopic surgery, any type of hemostatic procedure (injection, argon plasma coagulation, clipping), endoscopic resection, dilation, extraction of foreign bodies, percutaneous endoscopic jejunostomy, and implantation of self-expanding metal stents.[5,11–16] Enteroscopy techniques are also needed for investigations in the upper gastrointestinal tract in patients who require certain types of bariatric surgery, and for endoscopic retrograde cholangiopancreatography (ERCP) in patients with surgically altered anatomy.[17,18]

However, small bowel bleeding continues to be the main indication.[7,9,19] There is still a certain amount of confusion in the terminology used to define gastrointestinal bleeding. The terms overt and occult describe the type of bleeding; bleeding that is either macroscopically visible (melena, hematochezia) or macroscopically invisible; the latter can only be detected using stool tests. The term obscure refers to bleeding from an unclear location. Before nonsurgical enteroscopy was available, gastrointestinal bleeding was divided into upper gastrointestinal bleeding, in which the bleeding source was located proximal to the ligament of Treitz (duodenojejunal flexure); and lower gastrointestinal bleeding, in which the bleeding source was distal to the ligament of Treitz. Because the small bowel was unknown territory for endoscopists before the introduction of capsule endoscopy and DBE, the term obscure gastrointestinal bleeding was used as a synonym for suspected small bowel bleeding. Since the introduction of enteroscopy methods, the definition of gastrointestinal bleeding has had to be redefined, as shown in **Fig. 3**.[20] The term obscure should now be used for bleeding that remains unclear after a negative diagnostic work-up including small bowel endoscopy.

Appropriate patient selection and correct choice of the enteroscopy device to be used are mandatory for successful management of midgastrointestinal bleeding. For appropriate patient selection, information is required about the type of bleeding; its severity (with a potential need for blood transfusion); and the patient's medical history relative to anticoagulant medication, intake of nonsteroidal antiinflammatory drugs (NSAIDs), and prior abdominal surgery. The patient's age and concomitant diseases also need to be taken into account. Before any kind of enteroscopy is started, it is important to have a clear idea of the most likely cause of the bleeding and to take the appropriate decision about which kind of enteroscopy device is likely to be best in the situation. The same also applies to other indications for enteroscopy.

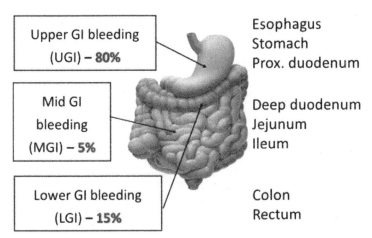

Fig. 3. The classification of different types of gastrointestinal (GI) bleeding. Prox., proximal.

In patients with chronic small bowel bleeding, the most common sources of bleeding are angiodysplasias, at least in Western countries. Argon plasma coagulation (APC) is therefore one of the most frequently used therapeutic methods. APC of angiodysplasias or vascular malformations is safe and effective, as various studies have shown.[12,21–26] Malignancies and any types of erosion or ulceration caused by NSAIDs, Crohn disease, large polyps, and ischemia in surgical anastomoses are other possible sources of bleeding that can lead to chronic MGIB.

In patients with acute ongoing MGIB, DBE or other enteroscopy techniques are the methods of choice, in view of their high diagnostic and therapeutic yield. The main sources of acute bleeding are angiodysplasias in patients who are receiving anticoagulant medication, Dieulafoy lesions, any type of ulceration, and the rare conditions of Meckel diverticulum or small bowel varices. In cases of severe bleeding, emergency DBE is challenging and should be performed by staff members with experience in emergency endoscopy and enteroscopy.

In recent years, Crohn disease has increasingly become the focus of interest. In patients with Crohn, enteroscopy is performed to detect ulcerations and stenoses (which may have been missed on radiographic imaging) and for decision making regarding the subsequent medical or surgical management. A higher risk of perforation during DBE was found in the group of patients with Crohn disease and steroid medication. This risk should be taken into account when performing DBE in this group of patients.[27–29]

Enteroscopy has also become important in patients with polyposis syndromes, because it provides the option of endoscopic resection in deeper parts of the small bowel without the need for surgery.[30–32]

All of the common indications for enteroscopy are described in detail in other articles in this issue. The remainder of this article explains why DBE is the most promising technique for managing small bowel diseases such as bleeding, Crohn disease, and polyposis syndromes.

Performance

DBE was first introduced in Japan by the technique's inventor, Hironori Yamamoto, in 2001 and in the Western hemisphere by our own group in 2003.[1,2] Thanks to technical developments and improvements, several double-balloon devices for different indications are now available (**Table 1**). The P type is the thinnest and its high flexibility allows deep insertion and complete enteroscopy in a high percentage of cases, even in

Table 1
Different double-balloon endoscopes and main areas of application

Scopes	EN-450P5	EN-450T5, EN-580T[a]	EC-450BI5, (EI-580 BT[a], Prototype)
Length (cm)	200	200	152
Diameter (mm)	8.5	9.4	9.4
Working Channel (mm)	2.2	2.8, 3.2[a]	2.8, 3.2[a]
Main Areas of Application	• Very deep/ complete enteroscopy • Difficult anatomy • Children	• Acute bleeding • Dilation • ERCP after altered anatomy with long loops • High resolution needed	• ERCP in surgically altered anatomy • Difficult ileocolonoscopy

[a] A larger working channel of 3.2 mm is available.

difficult anatomic conditions.[33,34] The T type has a slightly larger outer diameter, but consequently a larger working channel of 2.8 mm and 3.2 mm, respectively. The newer EN-580T device additionally provides easier handling for balloon insufflation and is a high-resolution endoscope (**Fig. 4**). The larger working channel makes the T type useful for cases of acute bleeding and for dilation, as well as ERCP in patients with surgically altered anatomy (if the double-balloon colonoscope is too short for access).[35] The double-balloon colonoscope can be recommended not only for difficult ileocolonoscopies but is also mainly used for ERCP in patients with surgically altered anatomy.[36,37] As a result of the reduced length of the colonoscope, all standard accessories for ERCP can be inserted, whereas for the longer T type only specially designed instruments can be used. The new prototype of a short double-balloon endoscope (EI-580BT, Fujifilm, Japan) provides high resolution, greater bending at the tip of the scope, and easier handling for balloon insufflation. For children, another prototype is being developed with an outer diameter of 7.7 mm and a working channel of 2.0 mm. The availability of different double-balloon endoscopes is a great advantage, because appropriate device selection is one of the key points for successful enteroscopy. For SBE and spiral enteroscopy, only 1 device and prototype is available.

DBE can be performed with the patients under sedoanalgetic medication. General anesthesia is only required in selected cases (eg, in children; in difficult procedures in younger patients, such as polypectomy of very large polyps; or in older patients with respiratory problems).[38]

In the early days of enteroscopy, bowel cleansing was only recommended for the anal approach. However, in the opinion and experience of the present author, preparation with a cleansing solution in cases of oral DBE can be recommended in patients with slow transit, oral iron substitution, prior abdominal surgery with Roux-en-Y reconstruction, and in those with signs of intestinal obstruction or when very deep insertion is planned. For the anal approach, patients should be prepared with split-dose cleansing as in colonoscopy.[39]

Outcome

Because DBE is the oldest technique for enteroscopy, there is considerable experience with the device and results from large databases are available.[23–26,29] The complication rates with diagnostic enteroscopy, at up to 1%, are higher than with diagnostic upper and lower gastrointestinal endoscopy. However, they are acceptable

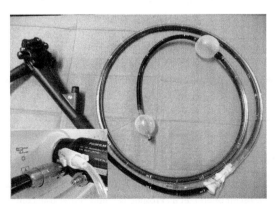

Fig. 4. The new-generation T-type double-balloon enteroscope (EN-580T). (*Courtesy* of Fujifilm Inc., Saitama, Japan)

because DBE is a much more complex investigation. As in conventional endoscopy, therapeutic interventions are associated with an overall complication rate of 3% to 4%, which is higher than with diagnostic procedures. Polypectomy of large polyps seems to be the intervention associated with the highest complication rate (up to 10%), especially during an endoscopist's learning period with the method.[11] The mortality is estimated at 0.05%.[24] Altogether, the complication rate and mortality are lower than with intraoperative enteroscopy, which has morbidity rates of 15% to 20% and mortality of up to 5%; DBE also requires fewer staff.[40,41] Intraoperative enteroscopy has consequently now become a method reserved for selected cases.

With appropriate patient selection, high diagnostic and therapeutic yields of 70% to 85% can be expected with DBE.[5,7,9] One reason for this may be the second balloon at the tip of the scope, which helps to stabilize the position and facilitates insertion even in difficult conditions. It may also be less traumatic. In addition, the balloon at the tip of the scope can also be inflated during withdrawal, so that it pulls apart the pleated folds and may lead to a reduced rate of missed lesions.

Another reason for the high yield is the high percentage of cases in which complete enteroscopy can be achieved if needed. The first prospective trial comparing the 1-balloon and 2-balloon techniques showed that DBE was associated with a rate of complete enteroscopy that was 3 times higher.[42] Complete enteroscopy is only required in approximately 20% of all patients. Achieving complete enteroscopy also represents an objective measure of the depth of insertion reached. Details are shown in **Table 2**. The comparative studies by Takano and colleagues[43] and Domagk and colleagues[44] presented contradictory results. Although the prospective single-center study in Japan confirmed that DBE has significantly better results in relation to complete enteroscopy, the European multicenter trial did not find a significant difference (**Table 3**). The problem with the latter trial was the generally very low rate of complete enteroscopy achieved, which was even less than the rate of 23% achieved in the German DBE registry.[24] Appropriate training when endoscopists are starting to practice enteroscopy, and ensuring a medium to high volume of investigations, are important for effective handling of enteroscopy. Skill is one of the key issues, as is shown by the author's own learning curve with an initial rate of complete enteroscopy of 45%, increasing up to approximately 90% within the following years.[7,45]

Compared with the manual form of spiral enteroscopy, DBE seems to allow deeper insertion, whereas spiral enteroscopy seems to be faster, at least in easy cases.[45–47] This contrast may change with the new motorized spiral enteroscope, but at present only a prototype of the device is available and clinical evaluation is still in progress.

Table 2
Results of a prospective comparative trial in Germany using the 1-balloon and 2-balloon techniques

	DBE (n = 50)	SBE (n = 50)	P Value
Preparation Time	10 min	6 min	<.0001
Investigation Time (Mean, Oral, and Anal)	80–90 min	75 min	<.0005
Diagnostic and Therapeutic Yield	72%	48%	<.025
Complete Enteroscopy	66%	22%	<.0001

From May A, Färber M, Aschmoneit I, et al. Prospective multicenter trial comparing push-and-pull enteroscopy with the single- and double-balloon techniques in patients with small-bowel disorders. Am J Gastroenterol 2010;105:575–81; with permission.

Table 3
Results of the prospective randomized Japanese and European trials on rates of complete enteroscopy with double-balloon endoscopy and single-balloon enteroscopy

	Complete Enteroscopy		
	DBE (%)	SBE (%)	P Value
Japanese Single-center Study[43]	57	0	<.0001
European Multicenter Trial[44]	18	11	NS

Abbreviation: NS, not significant.
    Data from Takano N, Yamdada A, Watabe H, et al. Single-balloon versus double-balloon endoscopy for achieving total enteroscopy: a randomized, controlled trial. Gastrointest Endosc 2011;73:734–9; and *Data from* Domagk D, Mensink P, Aktas H, et al. Single- vs. double-balloon enteroscopy in small-bowel diagnostics: a randomized multicenter trial. Endoscopy 2011;43:472–6.

SUMMARY

Since the introduction of DBE 15 years ago, flexible enteroscopy has become an established method in the diagnostic and therapeutic work-up of small bowel disorders. DBE is the first and thus the oldest technique for flexible enteroscopy without the need for a surgical approach. Considerable experience has been gained with the method in recent years, and most studies and publications on enteroscopy have been concerned with DBE. If appropriate patient selection is performed, high diagnostic and therapeutic yields of 70% to 85% can be expected with DBE. DBE also provides the highest rates of complete enteroscopy (up to 90%), which is needed in approximately 20% of all patients in whom enteroscopy is indicated. Achieving complete enteroscopy also represents an objective measure of the depth of insertion reached. The complication rates with diagnostic and therapeutic DBE can be estimated at approximately 1% and 3% to 4%, respectively. Polypectomy of large polyps seems to be the intervention associated with the highest complication rate, at up to 10%, especially during the learning period with the method. The mortality can be estimated at 0.05%.

Midgastrointestinal bleeding, Crohn disease, and polyposis syndromes are still the main indications for enteroscopy, but any type of small bowel disorder can be an indication. Since the introduction of enteroscopy methods, the classification of gastrointestinal bleeding has had to be redefined as involving upper gastrointestinal, midgastrointestinal, and lower gastrointestinal bleeding. The term obscure should now be used only for bleeding that remains unclear after a negative diagnostic work-up including small bowel endoscopy.

Appropriate patient selection, the correct choice of device, and skill are the key issues for successful enteroscopy. The availability of different double-balloon endoscopes is a great advantage, because it makes it possible to select suitable devices for any situation. Although carrying out enteroscopy has become easier because of technical developments and improvements, therapeutic interventions in the small bowel continue to be challenging, because of the thin wall of the small bowel and its high degree of vascularization.

REFERENCES

1. Yamamoto H, Sekine Y, Sato Y, et al. Total enteroscopy with a nonsurgical steerable double-balloon method. Gastrointest Endosc 2001;53:216–20.
2. May A, Nachbar L, Wardak A, et al. Double-balloon enteroscopy: preliminary experience in patients with obscure gastrointestinal bleeding or chronic abdominal pain. Endoscopy 2003;35:985–91.

3. Tsujikawa T, Saitoh Y, Andoh A, et al. Novel single-balloon enteroscopy for diagnosis and treatment of the small intestine: preliminary experiences. Endoscopy 2008;40:11–5.

4. Akerman P, Agrawal D, Cantero D, et al. Spiral enteroscopy with the new DSB overtube: a novel technique for deep peroral small bowel intubation. Endoscopy 2008;40:974–8.

5. Yamamoto H, Kita H, Sunada K, et al. Clinical outcomes of double-balloon endoscopy for the diagnosis and treatment of small-intestinal diseases. Clin Gastroenterol Hepatol 2004;2:1010–6.

6. Ell C, May A, Nachbar L, et al. Push-and-pull enteroscopy in the small bowel using the double-balloon technique: results of a prospective European multicenter study. Endoscopy 2005;37:613–6.

7. May A, Nachbar L, Ell C. Double-balloon enteroscopy (push-and-pull enteroscopy) of the small bowel: feasibility and diagnostic and therapeutic yield in patients with suspected small bowel disease. Gastrointest Endosc 2005;62:62–70.

8. Heine GD, Hadithi M, Groenen MJ, et al. Double-balloon enteroscopy: indications, diagnostic yield, and complications in a series of 275 patients with suspected small-bowel disease. Endoscopy 2006;38:42–8.

9. Zhong J, Ma T, Zhang C, et al. A retrospective study of the application on double-balloon enteroscopy in 378 patients with suspected small-bowel diseases. Endoscopy 2007;39:208–15.

10. Kuga R, Safatle-Ribeiro A, Ishida RK, et al. Small bowel endoscopy using the double-balloon technique: four-year results in a tertiary referral hospital in Brazil. Dig Dis 2008;26:318–23.

11. May A, Nachbar L, Pohl J, et al. Endoscopic interventions in the small bowel using double-balloon enteroscopy: feasibility and limitations. Am J Gastroenterol 2007;102:527–35.

12. May A, Friesing-Sosnik T, Manner H, et al. Long-term outcome after argon plasma coagulation of small-bowel lesions using double-balloon enteroscopy in patients with mid-gastrointestinal bleeding. Endoscopy 2011;43:759–65.

13. Despott EJ, Gupta A, Burling D, et al. Effective dilation of small-bowel strictures by double-balloon enteroscopy in patients with symptomatic Crohn's disease (with video). Gastrointest Endosc 2009;70(5):1030–6.

14. Sunada K, Shinozaki S, Nagayama M, et al. Long-term outcomes in patients with small intestinal strictures secondary to Crohn's disease after double-balloon endoscopy-assisted balloon dilation. Inflamm Bowel Dis 2016;22:380–6.

15. Despott EJ, Gabe S, Tripoli E, et al. Enteral access by double-balloon enteroscopy: an alternative method of direct percutaneous endoscopic jejunostomy placement. Dig Dis Sci 2011;56:494–8.

16. Ross AS, Semrad C, Waxman I, et al. Enteral stent placement by double balloon enteroscopy for palliation of malignant small bowel obstruction. Gastrointest Endosc 2006;64:835–7.

17. Tagaya N, Kasama K, Inamine S, et al. Evaluation of the excluded stomach by double-balloon endoscopy after laparoscopic Roux-en-Y gastric bypass. Obes Surg 2007;17:1165–70.

18. Raithel M, Dormann H, Naegel A, et al. Double-balloon-enteroscopy-based endoscopic retrograde cholangiopancreatography in post-surgical patients. World J Gastroenterol 2011;17:2302–14.

19. Xin L, Zhuan L, Yue-Ping J, et al. Indications, detectability, positive findings, total enteroscopy, and complications of diagnostic double-balloon enteroscopy: a systematic review of data over the first decade of use. Gastrointest Endosc 2011;74:563–70.

20. Ell C, May A. Mid-gastrointestinal bleeding: capsule endoscopy and push-and-pull enteroscopy give rise to a new medical term. Endoscopy 2006;38:73–5.

21. Gerson LB, Batenic MA, Newsom SL, et al. Long-term outcomes after double-balloon enteroscopy for obscure gastrointestinal bleeding. Clin Gastroenterol Hepatol 2009;7:664–9.

22. Shinozaki S, Yamamoto H, Yano T, et al. Favorable long-term outcomes of repeat endotherapy for small-intestine vascular lesions by double-balloon endoscopy. Gastrointest Endosc 2014;80:112–7.

23. Mensink PB, Haringsma J, Kucharzik T, et al. Complications of double balloon enteroscopy: a multicenter survey. Endoscopy 2007;39:613–5.

24. Möschler O, May AD, Müller MK, et al. Complications in double-balloon enteroscopy: results of the German DBE register. Z Gastroenterol 2008;46:266–70 [in German].

25. Gerson L, Tokar J, Chiorean M, et al. Complications associated with double balloon enteroscopy at nine US centers. Clin Gastroenterol Hepatol 2009;7:1177–82.

26. Moschler O, May A, Muller MK, et al. Complications in and performance of double-balloon enteroscopy (DBE): results from a large prospective DBE database in Germany. Endoscopy 2011;43:484–9.

27. Takenaka K, Ohtsuka K, Kitazume Y, et al. Comparison of magnetic resonance and balloon enteroscopic examination of the small intestine in patients with Crohn's disease. Gastroenterology 2014;147:334–42.

28. Rahman A, Ross A, Leighton JA, et al. Double-balloon enteroscopy in Crohn's disease: findings and impact on management in a multicenter retrospective study. Gastrointest Endosc 2015;82:102–7.

29. Odagiri H, Matsui H, Fushimi K, et al. Factors associated with perforation related to diagnostic balloon-assisted enteroscopy: analysis of a national inpatient database in Japan. Endoscopy 2015;47:143–6.

30. Plum N, May AD, Manner H, et al. Peutz-Jeghers syndrome: endoscopic detection and treatment of small bowel polyps by double-balloon enteroscopy. Z Gastroenterol 2007;45:1049–55.

31. Gorospe EC, Alexander JA, Bruining DH, et al. Performance of double-balloon enteroscopy for the management of small bowel polyps in hamartomatous polyposis syndromes. J Gastroenterol Hepatol 2013;28(2):268–73.

32. Serrano M, Mão-de-Ferro S, Pinho R, et al. Double-balloon enteroscopy in the management of patients with Peutz-Jeghers syndrome: a retrospective cohort multicenter study. Rev Esp Enferm Dig 2013;105:594–9.

33. Teshima CW, Aktas H, van Buuren HR, et al. Retrograde double balloon enteroscopy: comparing performance of solely versus combined same-day anterograde and retrograde procedure. Scand J Gastroenterol 2011;36:220–6.

34. Murino A, Nakamura M, Despott EJ, et al. Factors associated with reduced insertion depth at double balloon enteroscopy: a retrospective, multivariate analysis. Dig Liver Dis 2014;46(10):956–8.

35. Kawashima H, Nakamura M, Ohno E, et al. Impact of instrument channel diameter on therapeutic endoscopic retrograde cholangiography using balloon-assisted enteroscopy. Dig Endosc 2014;26(Suppl 2):127–9.

36. Siddiqui AA, Chaaya A, Shelton C, et al. Utility of the short double-balloon enteroscope to perform pancreaticobiliary interventions in patients with surgically altered anatomy in a US multicenter study. Dig Dis Sci 2013;58:858–64.

37. Tsutsumi K, Kato H, Muro S, et al. ERCP using a short double-balloon enteroscope in patients with prior pancreatoduodenectomy: higher maneuverability supplied by the efferent-limb route. Surg Endosc 2015;29:1944–51.

38. Tanaka S, Mitsui K, Tatsuguchi A, et al. Current status of double-balloon endoscopy-indications, insertion rout, sedation, complications, technical matters. Gastrointest Endosc 2007;66(3 Suppl):S30–3.
39. Radaelli F, Paggi S, Hassan C, et al. Split-dose preparation for colonoscopy increases adenoma detection rate: a randomised controlled trial in an organised screening programme. Gut 2015. [Epub ahead of print].
40. Hartmann D, Schmidt H, Bolz G, et al. A prospective two-center study comparing wireless capsule endoscopy with intraoperative enteroscopy in patients with obscure GI bleeding. Gastrointest Endosc 2005;61:826–32.
41. Bonnet S, Douard R, Malamut G, et al. Intraoperative enteroscopy in the management of obscure gastrointestinal bleeding. Dig Liver Dis 2013;45:277–84.
42. May A, Färber M, Aschmoneit I, et al. Prospective multicenter trial comparing push-and-pull enteroscopy with the single- and double-balloon techniques in patients with small-bowel disorders. Am J Gastroenterol 2010;105:575–81.
43. Takano N, Yamdada A, Watabe H, et al. Single-balloon versus double-balloon endoscopy for achieving total enteroscopy: a randomized, controlled trial. Gastrointest Endosc 2011;73:734–9.
44. Domagk D, Mensink P, Aktas H, et al. Single- vs. double-balloon enteroscopy in small-bowel diagnostics: a randomized multicenter trial. Endoscopy 2011;43:472–6.
45. Messer I, May A, Manner H, et al. Prospective, randomized, single-center trial comparing double-balloon enteroscopy and spiral enteroscopy in patients with suspected small-bowel disorders. Gastrointest Endosc 2013;77:241–9.
46. May A, Manner H, Aschmoneit I, et al. Prospective, cross-over, single-center trial comparing oral double-balloon enteroscopy and oral spiral enteroscopy in patients with suspected small-bowel vascular malformations. Endoscopy 2011;43:477–83.
47. Despott EJ, Murino A, Bourikas L, et al. A prospective comparison of performance during back-to-back, anterograde manual spiral enteroscopy and double-balloon enteroscopy. Dig Liver Dis 2015;47:395–400.

Single-Balloon Enteroscopy

Philipp Lenz, MD[a], Dirk Domagk, MD[b],*

KEYWORDS

- Small-bowel endoscopy • Single-balloon enteroscopy
- Balloon-assisted enteroscopy • Device-assisted enteroscopy • Carbon dioxide
- Diagnostic yield • Complete enteroscopy rate

KEY POINTS

- Single-balloon enteroscopy and double-balloon enteroscopy are equally suitable for small bowel exploration.
- The individual learning curve should be comprised of about 30 examinations for experienced endoscopists.
- Carbon dioxide should be used as insufflation gas for single-balloon endoscopy procedures.

INTRODUCTION

With the beginning of the millennium, wireless video capsule endoscope (VCE) and double-balloon enteroscopy (DBE) were introduced.[1,2] Both devices allowed the investigation of the small bowel for the first time, the latter one not only as diagnostic modality, but also with the option to perform therapeutic interventions (EN-450T5, Fujinon Incorporated, Saitama, Japan).

Several years later, the single-balloon enteroscope (SBE) appeared on the market.[3,4] This newly introduced balloon-assisted enteroscopy device (SIF-Q180, Olympus Optical, Tokyo, Japan) has only 1 balloon, located on the tip of the overtube. By this means, the set-up of the system is facilitated, which shortens preparation time. A recent Pubmed search demonstrated approximately 1071 published studies using DBE, and 321 with an SBE. An ongoing debate includes the different panenteroscopy rates of both systems and the diagnostic impact of complete visualization of the small bowel.[5–9]

Disclosure: The authors have nothing to disclose.
[a] Department of Palliative Care, Institute of Palliative Care, University Hospital of Muenster, Albert-Schweitzer-Campus 1, Building W30, Muenster 48149, Germany; [b] Department of Medicine I, Josephs-Hospital Warendorf, Academic Teaching Hospital, University of Muenster, Am Krankenhaus 2, Warendorf 48231, Germany
* Corresponding author.
E-mail address: domagkd@uni-muenster.de

Gastrointest Endoscopy Clin N Am 27 (2017) 123–131
http://dx.doi.org/10.1016/j.giec.2016.08.007

The next new kid on the block, the spiral enteroscope (SE, Endo-Ease Discovery SB, Spirus Medical, Stoughton, Massachusetts), promised to offer the most stable position in the small bowel, and, therefore, to be especially suitable for therapeutic interventions.[10] To date, approximately 82 citations in Pubmed using SE are available. Currently, a new motorized version of the spiral enteroscope is being tested and may change the importance of this enteroscopy device.

In a line with all the other authors and experts of enteroscopy within this journal, this article will aim to describe the possibilities and limitations of single-balloon enteroscopy. Additionally, the article will compare the performance of the SBE with DBE and SE, not on a personal, eminence-based judgment, but on the basis of randomized controlled trials (RCTs).

SINGLE-BALLOON ENDOSCOPY FOR EVALUATION OF THE SMALL BOWEL

As balloon-assisted enteroscopy system, the SBE (SIF-Q180, Olympus Optical, Tokyo, Japan) consists of a standard endoscope back-loaded with an overtube equipped with a balloon at its distal end (**Fig. 1**). The rigid overtube is supposed to avoid looping of the bowel and to direct the pushing forces directly to the tip of the endoscope to advance the enteroscope into the deep small bowel. The inflated balloon is supposed to fix the intestine to the endoscope system. In contrast to the DBE system, the SBE uses the angulated tip of the endoscope (hooked-tip) to fix the intestine to the scope.[3,4] Technically, there are 2 options to push the endoscope deeper into the small bowel[3]:

1. Conventional push-and-pull-technique: the enteroscope and the overtube are pulled back in order to shrink and straighten the bowel; the tip of the endoscope is further threaded into the small bowel
2. Simultaneous push-and-pull technique: the inflated overtube is pulled back, whereas the enteroscope is pushed forward simultaneously

Usually complete small bowel visualization may be accomplished by a combined oral and anal approach.[11]

Insertion Depth

With respect to the literature and to the authors' own experience, most endoscopists seem to estimate intubation depth during enteroscopy according to the method

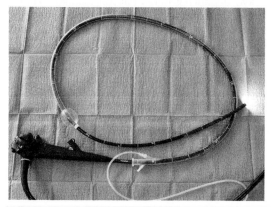

Fig. 1. The single-balloon enteroscope (SIF-Q180, Olympus Medical Systems Corp, Tokyo, Japan) consists of a standard endoscope back-loaded with an overtube equipped with a balloon at its distal end.

described by May and colleagues.[12] By this method, endoscopists assess the efficacy of each push-and-pull maneuver and document the advancement in centimeters on a standardized sheet. The sum of the recorded numbers at the end of the examination estimates the length of the small intestine that has been successfully visualized. Another method published by Li and colleagues[13] offers an alternative option to estimate intubation depth by calculating the overtube advancement (5 cm overtube = 40 cm small bowel). Efthymiou and colleagues[14] proposed fold counts on withdrawal of the enteroscope to have good correlation with measured intubation depth, providing a further simple alternative to existing methods.

Diagnostic Yield

If the endoscopic method enables the clinician to confirm or rule out a diagnosis, one has a positive diagnostic yield. Usually, diagnostic yield improves over the course of time for 2 reasons:

1. Learning curve: endoscopists improve their skills using a new endoscopy device[11,15–17]
2. At introduction of new endoscopic modalities, selection of patients being investigated by this method is often unfiltered; indications for examining patients are not strict and are less focused, resulting, consequently, in a lower diagnostic yield[18]

Carbon Dioxide Versus Air Insufflation

Gastrointestinal (GI) endoscopy applying air for insufflation is not an excellent solution, because, after the procedure, large amounts of air remain trapped in the bowel segments that were inspected.[19,20] The insufflated air has to pass through the remaining GI tract and exits via naturalis through the anus. Thus, abdominal pain and discomfort during and after endoscopy due to retention of air are often observed.[21–23] Due to this clear disadvantage, alternative gases are needed for insufflation during endoscopy. In contrast to air, carbon dioxide (CO_2) is rapidly absorbed from the bowel; large amounts of CO_2 can be incorporated within minutes from the GI tract and may subsequently be exhaled. In several studies, CO_2 as insufflation gas resulted in more comfortable examinations in both colonoscopy and flexible sigmoidoscopy; CO_2 insufflation significantly reduced procedure-related pain and discomfort.[21–23] Although the advantage of CO_2 has also been shown in several other studies,[24–28] air is still most commonly used for bowel distension in investigations of the large bowel.[29]

Enteroscopy of the small bowel is an endoscopic technique with comparatively long investigation times (75 minutes in average).[30] Therefore, large amounts of gas often have to be insufflated, leading to an extensive distension of the small bowel during and after the endoscopic examination. In an RCT, the authors were to show that the use of CO_2 at DBE does not only reduce the peri-interventional pain, but leads also to deeper intubation of the small bowel. Furthermore, a reduced need for sedation drugs was recorded in the CO_2 group, in contrast to the patients receiving air as insufflation gas[30]; these results were confirmed by another working group.[31] Analogous to DBE, Li and colleagues[32] reported both reduced sedating drugs and improved intubation depths also for single balloon enteroscopy, on average about 90 cm more than the control group.

Whereas in previous studies for DBE[30,31] and also in the trial by Li and colleagues[32] (for SBE), the use of CO_2 significantly improved oral insertion depths, in the authors' study of SBE, this improvement was not observed for all patients in the CO_2 group.[33] In the subgroup analysis of patients with a history of abdominal surgery, the use of CO_2 insufflation appeared to be particularly beneficial, as oral insertion depth was

Table 1
Randomized controlled trials for DAE (including single-balloon endoscopy)

Investigated Procedures (Citation)	Study Design/Population RCT/CS/RS	n/(month)	Depth of Insertion, cm, Mean ± standard deviation (SD) or Range Oral (Antegrad)	Anal (Retrograde)	Combined	Procedure Characteristics Complete Small-Bowel Visual x/yᵃ (%)	Insufflation (gas)	Procedure Time (mean ± SD or range, min)	Preparation Time (total, min)	Diagnostic Yield (%)	Therapeutic Procedures (%)	AE (SAE) (%)
SBE (Olympus) vs	RCT	130/(12)	258 (100–560)	118 (5–300)	373 (100–620)	7/65 (11%)	CO$_2$	96 (35–135)	—	37	5	0 (0)
DBE (Fujinon) (Domagk et al 2011)[11]			253 (120–450)	107 (10–250)	360 (180–550)	12/65 (18%)		105 (40–140)		43	9	
SBE (Olympus) vs	RCT	38/(24)	—	—	—	0/18 (0%)	—	Oral: 92.8 ± 20.6 Anal: 93.1 ± 22.6	—	61.1	11.1	0 (0)
DBE (Fujinon) (Takano et al 2011)[35]						8/20 (57%)ᵇ		Oral: 70.4 ± 26.5 Anal: 90.4 ± 13.7		50.0	15.0	

Technique	Design	No./(AE)			Mean depth (cm)		Insufflation	Procedure time (min)		Diagnostic yield (%)	Therapeutic (%)	Complete enteroscopy	SAE
SBE (Fujinon) vs	RCT	100/(13)	—	—	203.8 cm	72.1 cm	Air	(Fujinon): Oral 54 (23–90); Anal 60 (20–100)	(Fujinon): Oral 6 (4–10); Anal 6 (3–15)	(Fujinon): 42	(Fujinon): 48	(Fujinon): 11/50 (22%)	3 (0)
DBE (Fujinon) (May et al 2010)[16]					234.1 cm (P = .176)	75.2 cm (P = .835)		(Oral): Oral 67 (38–100)[b] Anal: 62 (22–115)	Oral: 10 (5–15)[b] Anal: 10 (5–20)	52	72[b]	33/50 (66%)[b]	—
SBE (Olympus) vs	RCT	119/(24)	—	—			Air	60 min	—	57	32		
DBE (Fujinon) (Efthymiou et al 2012)[14]								60 min		53 (P = .697)	26		—

Abbreviations: —, not defined; AE, adverse events; APC, argon-plasma coagulation; CD, Crohn disease; CE, capsule endoscopy; CS, case control study or case series; GA, general anesthesia; P, prospective; RCT, randomized controlled trials; RS, retrospective study; SAE, severe adverse events.
[a] Complete small bowel visualization attempted (y) and successful (x).
[b] Significant difference (P<.05).

Data from May A, Manner H, Aschmoneit I, et al. Prospective, cross-over, single-center trial comparing oral double-balloon enteroscopy and oral spiral enteroscopy in patients with suspected small-bowel vascular malformations. Endoscopy 2011;43:477–83; and Efthymiou M, Desmond PV, Brown G, et al. SINGLE-01: a randomized, controlled trial comparing the efficacy and depth of insertion of single- and double-balloon enteroscopy by using a novel method to determine insertion depth. Gastrointest Endosc 2012;76:972–80.

significantly greater within the CO_2 group (about 60 cm more than in the air group). Because the development or existence of intraperitoneal adhesions after abdominal surgery may still be a relevant clinical problem,[34] the use of CO_2 with its favorable characteristics (particularly rapid intestinal absorption) might have its impact, especially in patients with previous abdominal surgery.[33]

Single- Versus Double-Balloon Endoscopy

In 2011, the authors published the first head-to-head comparison trial of Fujinon's DBE (EN-450T5) versus Olympus' SBE (SIF-Q180).[11] Noninferiority was shown with respect to the insertion depths. With regard to complete visualization, the authors could not show noninferiority; whether SBE is inferior, equivalent, or even superior compared with DBE remains an open question. Diagnostic yield, rate of complications between the 2 systems, and patient discomfort scores during and after the procedures were comparable.[11]

Up to now, 4 RCTs have been published that compare the DBE and SBE techniques,[11,14,16,35] of which 3 RCTs compared the device-assisted enteroscopy (DAE) systems.[11,14,35] According to the published data and review on the so far established DAE systems,[36] the DBE and the SBE systems have similar procedural characteristics (eg, diagnostic yield, therapeutic interventions, adverse events).

Significance of Complete Enteroscopy Rates

The impact of complete endoscopic evaluation of the small bowel in studies has been a matter of long and intense discussions throughout the endoscopy community at scientific conferences and in literature.[5–7,37] According to the literature, the rate of complete endoscopy differs tremendously, between 18% and 66% in larger studies. However, what often remains unclear at first sight is whether complete enteroscopy was attempted at all in these studies. Whenever a pathologic finding (eg, bleeding source, neoplasia, inflammation) is identified, many endoscopist would be satisfied with the diagnostic/therapeutic result of the examination. Consequently, in many studies, these cases might have been mixed, presenting a heterogenous group of patients. Other factors include a history of previous abdominal surgery, different distribution (of positive findings) in Eastern and Western countries,[14,38] or different methods for calculating complete endoscopic response (achieved vs attempted or achieved vs whole-study population).[6] Nevertheless, the clinical importance of complete endoscopic response remains controversial. In the authors' opinion, the most important factor for evaluating clinical relevance is the diagnostic yield.[36] With respect to DBE and the SBE, both systems have never shown any differences with regard to diagnostic yield, leading to the conclusion that both systems are equally suitable in daily general gastroenterology practice[7] (**Table 1**).

SINGLE-BALLOON ENDOSCOPY VERSUS THE SPIRAL ENDOSCOPE

Up to now, no RCT testing SBE versus SE has existed. Only 1 retrospective analysis evaluates the procedural performance of both endoscopic devices.[39] No significant difference was found in diagnostic yield of SE compared with SBE (43.4% vs 59.6%, $P = .12$), although the insertion depth was significantly higher in the SE group (301 cm vs 222 cm; $P = .001$).[39]

SUMMARY

SBE is a safe diagnostic tool to evaluate and screen for intestinal disorders. Compared with all other device-assisted enteroscopy modalities (SE, DBE), the diagnostic yield showed no difference, indicating that it is equally suitable for gastroenterologist in daily clinical routine.[7] The enteroscope system of choice should depend on the endoscopist's personal experience with the different providers on the market. With respect to the different handling of the devices (1 vs 2 balloons vs spiral), the authors recommended testing the different enteroscopes in action before coming to a decision for a certain DAE system.

With regard to the aspect of the learning curve, the authors propose defining a special curriculum to improve diagnostic yield and quality. The authors' single-center experience gives the impression that a frequent change in investigators could have a negative impact on procedural characteristics.[18]

To summarize, balloon-assisted enteroscopy is a strenuous and time-consuming investigation. To meet a certain claim in diagnostic quality, enteroscopy should remain a part of the advanced endoscopy teaching curriculum.

REFERENCES

1. Iddan G, Meron G, Glukhovsky A, et al. Wireless capsule endoscopy. Nature 2000;405:417.
2. Yamamoto H, Sekine Y, Sato Y, et al. Total enteroscopy with a nonsurgical steerable double-balloon method. Gastrointest Endosc 2001;53:216–20.
3. Hartmann D, Eickhoff A, Tamm R, et al. Balloon-assisted enteroscopy using a single-balloon technique. Endoscopy 2007;39(Suppl 1):E276.
4. Tsujikawa T, Saitoh Y, Andoh A, et al. Novel single-balloon enteroscopy for diagnosis and treatment of the small intestine: preliminary experiences. Endoscopy 2008;40:11–5.
5. May A. How much importance do we have to place on complete enteroscopy? Gastrointest Endosc 2010;73:740–2.
6. Xin L, Gao Y, Liao Z, et al. The reasonable calculation of complete enteroscopy rate for balloon-assisted enteroscopy. Endoscopy 2011;43:832.
7. Lenz P, Domagk D, Mensink P, et al. Single- versus double-balloon enteroscopy: the evidence base. Endoscopy 2012;44:799.
8. May A. Small-bowel endoscopy. Endoscopy 2012;44:375–7.
9. Manno M, Barbera C, Bertani H, et al. Double- vs. single-balloon enteroscopy: and the winner is. Endoscopy 2012;44:883.
10. Akerman PA, Agrawal D, Cantero D, et al. Spiral enteroscopy with the new DSB overtube: a novel technique for deep peroral small-bowel intubation. Endoscopy 2008;40:974–8.
11. Domagk D, Mensink P, Aktas H, et al. Single- vs. double-balloon enteroscopy in small-bowel diagnostics: a randomized multicenter trial. Endoscopy 2011;43:472–6.
12. May A, Nachbar L, Schneider M, et al. Push-and-pull enteroscopy using the double-balloon technique: method of assessing depth of insertion and training of the enteroscopy technique using the Erlangen Endo-Trainer. Endoscopy 2005;37:66–70.
13. Li XB, Dai J, Chen HM, et al. A novel modality for the estimation of the enteroscope insertion depth during double-balloon enteroscopy. Gastrointest Endosc 2010;72:999–1005.
14. Efthymiou M, Desmond PV, Brown G, et al. SINGLE-01: a randomized, controlled trial comparing the efficacy and depth of insertion of single- and double-balloon enteroscopy by using a novel method to determine insertion depth. Gastrointest Endosc 2012;76:972–80.

15. Gross SA, Stark ME. Initial experience with double-balloon enteroscopy at a U.S. center. Gastrointest Endosc 2008;67:890–7.

16. May A, Färber M, Aschmoneit I, et al. Prospective multicenter trial comparing push-and-pull enteroscopy with the single- and double-balloon techniques in patients with small-bowel disorders. Am J Gastroenterol 2010;105:575–81.

17. Mehdizadeh S, Ross A, Gerson L, et al. What is the learning curve associated with double-balloon enteroscopy? Technical details and early experience in 6 U.S. tertiary care centers. Gastrointest Endosc 2006;64:740–50.

18. Lenz P, Roggel M, Domagk D. Double- vs. single-balloon enteroscopy: single center experience with emphasis on procedural performance. Int J Colorectal Dis 2013;28:1239–46.

19. Bretthauer M, Hoff GS, Thiis-Evensen E, et al. Air and carbon dioxide volumes insufflated during colonoscopy. Gastrointest Endosc 2003;58:203–6.

20. Hussein AM, Bartram CI, Williams CB. Carbon dioxide insufflation for more comfortable colonoscopy. Gastrointest Endosc 1984;30:68–70.

21. Bretthauer M, Thiis-Evensen E, Huppertz-Hauss G, et al. NORCCAP (Norwegian colorectal cancer prevention): a randomised trial to assess the safety and efficacy of carbon dioxide versus air insufflation in colonoscopy. Gut 2002;50:604–7.

22. Stevenson GW, Wilson JA, Wilkinson J, et al. Pain following colonoscopy: elimination with carbon dioxide. Gastrointest Endosc 1992;38:564–7.

23. Sumanac K, Zealley I, Fox BM, et al. Minimizing postcolonoscopy abdominal pain by using CO_2 insufflation: a prospective, randomized, double blind, controlled trial evaluating a new commercially available CO_2 delivery system. Gastrointest Endosc 2002;56:190–4.

24. Bretthauer M, Hoff G, Thiis-Evensen E, et al. Carbon dioxide insufflation reduces discomfort due to flexible sigmoidoscopy in colorectal cancer screening. Scand J Gastroenterol 2002;37:1103–7.

25. Bretthauer M, Lynge AB, Thiis-Evensen E, et al. Carbon dioxide insufflation in colonoscopy: safe and effective in sedated patients. Endoscopy 2005;37:706–9.

26. Bretthauer M, Seip B, Aasen S, et al. Carbon dioxide insufflation for more comfortable endoscopic retrograde cholangiopancreatography: a randomized, controlled, double-blind trial. Endoscopy 2007;39:58–64.

27. Riss S, Akan B, Mikola B, et al. CO_2 insufflation during colonoscopy decreases post-interventional pain in deeply sedated patients: a randomized controlled trial. Wien Klin Wochenschr 2009;121:464–8.

28. Wong JC, Yau KK, Cheung HY, et al. Towards painless colonoscopy: a randomized controlled trial on carbon dioxide-insufflating colonoscopy. ANZ J Surg 2008;78:871–4.

29. Janssens F, Deviere J, Eisendrath P, et al. Carbon dioxide for gut distension during digestive endoscopy: technique and practice survey. World J Gastroenterol 2009;15:1475–9.

30. Domagk D, Bretthauer M, Lenz P, et al. Carbon dioxide insufflation improves intubation depth in double-balloon enteroscopy: a randomized, controlled, double-blind trial. Endoscopy 2007;39:1064–7.

31. Hirai F, Beppu T, Nishimura T, et al. Carbon dioxide insufflation compared with air insufflation in double-balloon enteroscopy: a prospective, randomized, double-blind trial. Gastrointest Endosc 2011;73:743–9.

32. Li X, Zhao YJ, Dai J, et al. Carbon dioxide insufflation improves the intubation depth and complete enteroscopy rate in single-balloon enteroscopy: a randomised, controlled, double-blind trial. Gut 2014;63:1560–5.

33. Lenz P, Meister T, Manno M, et al. CO_2 insufflation during single-balloon entero-scopy: a multicenter randomized controlled trial. Endoscopy 2014;46:53–8.

34. Brochhausen C, Schmitt VH, Planck CN, et al. Current strategies and future per-spectives for intraperitoneal adhesion prevention. J Gastrointest Surg 2012;16:1256–74.

35. Takano N, Yamada A, Watabe H, et al. Single-balloon versus double-balloon endoscopy for achieving complete enteroscopy: a randomized, controlled trial. Gastrointest Endosc 2011;73:734–9.

36. Lenz P, Domagk D. Double- vs. single-balloon vs. spiral enteroscopy. Best Pract Res Clin Gastroenterol 2012;26:303–13.

37. Moreels TG. Device-assisted enteroscopy: how deep is deep enteroscopy? Gas-trointest Endosc 2012;76:981–2.

38. Xin L, Liao Z, Jiang YP, et al. Indications, detectability, positive findings, complete enteroscopy, and complications of diagnostic double-balloon endoscopy: a sys-tematic review of data over the first decade of use. Gastrointest Endosc 2011;74:563–70.

39. Khashab MA, Lennon AM, Dunbar KB, et al. A comparative evaluation of single-balloon enteroscopy and spiral enteroscopy for patients with mid-gut disorders. Gastrointest Endosc 2010;72:766–72.

Small Bowel Imaging

Computed Tomography Enterography, Magnetic Resonance Enterography, Angiography, and Nuclear Medicine

Jeff L. Fidler, MD*, Ajit H. Goenka, MD, Chad J. Fleming, MD,
James C. Andrews, MD

KEYWORDS

- CT enterography • MR enterography • Angiography • PET/MRI • Crohn disease
- GI bleeding

KEY POINTS

- The computed tomography enterography (CTE) radiation dose has significantly decreased over the last several years.
- CTE has superior temporal and spatial resolution, and routinely higher image quality compared with magnetic resonance enterography (MRE).
- MRE should be considered the cross-sectional imaging study of choice for the surveillance of Crohn disease if high-quality examinations can be obtained.
- Catheter angiography is useful in the evaluation of vascular disease such as vasculitis, evaluation of patients with chronic gastrointestinal (GI) hemorrhage, treatment of acute GI hemorrhage, guidance for surgical resection of small bowel disease, and in the evaluation and treatment of the mesenteric venous system.
- Hybrid imaging techniques incorporating radionuclide imaging show promising results for evaluating small bowel bleeding and Crohn disease and may play a larger role in the future.

INTRODUCTION

Radiology examinations play a major role in the diagnosis, management, and surveillance of diseases of the small bowel and are complementary to endoscopic techniques. Advances in technology have translated into improved performance that has led to more widespread implementation of imaging for suspected small bowel disease. Computed tomography enterography (CTE) and magnetic resonance enterography (MRE) are now the cross-sectional imaging studies of choice for many small bowel

Disclosures: None.
Department of Radiology, Mayo Clinic, 200 First Street SW, Rochester, MN 55905, USA
* Corresponding author.
E-mail address: fidler.jeff@mayo.edu

Gastrointest Endoscopy Clin N Am 27 (2017) 133–152
http://dx.doi.org/10.1016/J.giec.2016.08.008
1052-5157/17/© 2016 Elsevier Inc. All rights reserved.

diseases. Catheter angiography still plays an important role in the evaluation and treatment of vascular abnormalities. New developments in radionuclide imaging, including the emergence of hybrid imaging techniques, have shown promise for the evaluation of small bowel bleeding and Crohn disease and may play a larger role in the future. This article reviews recent advances in technology, diagnosis, and therapeutic options for selected small bowel disorders. It is beyond the scope of this article to go into detail on many of these topics and several excellent references and reviews are included for further reading.

COMPUTED TOMOGRAPHY ENTEROGRAPHY AND MAGNETIC RESONANCE ENTEROGRAPHY
Advantages, Limitations, and Technical Advances

CTE and MRE are cross-sectional imaging techniques that are optimized for imaging of the small bowel. Each technique has advantages and limitations that make it better suited for certain clinical indications and scenarios (**Table 1**).

Advantages of CTE include higher spatial resolution that can improve detection of small subtle abnormalities such as small masses and vascular abnormalities. CTE is widely available and fast. Images of the entire abdomen and pelvis can be obtained in one breath hold. This leads to better patient tolerance with less motion artifact and more routinely higher quality examinations.

The main advantage of MRE is the ability to image the small bowel without radiation exposure. This is helpful in patients who are younger or need surveillance of

Table 1
Advantages and limitations of computed tomography enterography and magnetic resonance enterography

	CTE	MRE
Resolution	2–3 mm	3–5 mm
# phases	Few	Many
Quality	Better	Variable
Tolerability	Better	Less
Scan time	1 breath hold	35–45 min (breath holds)
Interpretation	Requires less expertise	Requires more expertise More variable
Evaluation of other organs	Excellent	More limited May require additional studies
Costs	—	More expensive
Access	Better May be easier to schedule	—
Risks	Radiation Intravenous contrast	Safer intravenous contrast Brain deposition of contrast (uncertain risk)
Bowel contrast	May obscure abnormalities Contrast based on indication Neutral contrast to detect hyperenhancing lesions Positive contrast to detect isodense lesions	Most agents biphasic Less chance of obscuration
Soft tissue contrast	—	Better

abnormalities such as inflammatory bowel disease (IBD) and polyposis syndromes. MRE also has superior soft tissue contrast; therefore, some abnormalities and enhancing areas may be more conspicuous. MRE also has the ability to perform multiple different pulse sequences, each with unique properties and information. Multiphasic imaging can be performed, demonstrating bowel peristalsis and physiology that may be altered in certain conditions. MRE also is more informative than CTE when intravenous contrast cannot be administered.

The main limitation of CTE is radiation exposure. Over the last several years, improvements in computed tomography (CT) technology have allowed the dose for CTE to be decreased significantly. By using lower voltage (kVp) and automatic tube current modulation with noise-reduction algorithms, the radiation dose has been reduced from 15 to 20 mGy to less than 10 mGy; doses less than 5 mGy have been reported (**Fig. 1**).[1] Studies have shown no significant decrease in performance in detecting high-contrast hyperenhancing lesions such as Crohn disease when using these lower dose techniques.[2,3] However, the detection of lower contrast hypoattenuating lesions in certain organs may be compromised.

Limitations of MRE include access and costs. MRE examinations typically are much longer (35–45 minutes) and require multiple breath holds that can lead to patient tiring, motion artifacts, and suboptimal image quality. MRE is optimized for imaging of the small bowel and, therefore, dedicated high-resolution imaging of other organs such as the bile ducts may not be possible in a single examination. For example, a dedicated MR cholangiopancreatography may need to be performed to evaluate for primary sclerosing cholangitis.

Oral Contrast

Ingestion of large volumes (900–1500 mL) of oral contrast agents is necessary to distend the bowel for both CT and MRE. Several agents have been evaluated. Currently, the most widely used agent in the United States is a low concentration barium agent (VoLumen, Bracco) that appears near water density on CT and improves

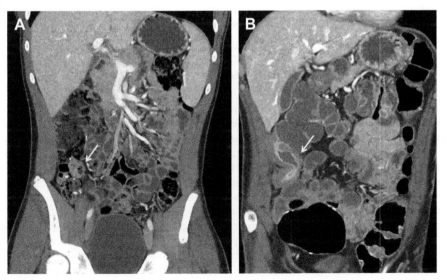

Fig. 1. Low-dose CTE performed with an estimated dose of 3 mSv (*A*) and 4 mSv (*B*) in 2 separate patients with Crohn ileitis (*arrows*).

detection of hyperenhancing abnormalities. This agent can also be used for MRE. However, current agents may not be well tolerated by patients. This may lead to decreased ingestion and bowel distention, requiring a dedicated enteroclysis or the placement of a nasogastric tube to administer the contrast into the stomach. A new flavoring agent for CT has been evaluated for enterography and may be better tolerated by patients.[4]

Oral contrast agents are classified according to their imaging characteristics on CT and MR. On CT, neutral agents have a density near water and positive agents have high density. On MR, agents can be negative (low signal on T1- and T2-weighted images), positive (high signal on T1- and T2-weighted images), or biphasic (low signal on T1- and high signal on T2-weighted images). Each agent has advantages and limitations. A limitation of CTE is the need to decide which type of oral contrast agent should be administered. For most CTE examinations, a neutral contrast agent is administered. The density of neutral agents is similar to water and allows improved detection of hyperenhancing lesions. However, if the bowel is not well distended, lesions that enhance to the same density as the bowel wall (isodense) may be missed. Positive contrast agents have a higher density and allow improved visualization of isodense lesions in poorly distended bowel but may obscure detection of hyperenhancing lesions such as carcinoid tumors, vascular lesions, and active bleeding. Most MR oral contrast agents have biphasic characteristics and are low-signal intensity on T1-weighted images and high-signal intensity on T2-weighted images. These MR signal characteristics reduce the likelihood of obscuring a lesion.

Enteroclysis

CT and MRE examinations are only performed at a limited number of institutions because of their complexity. These examinations require placement of a nasoenteric tube with administration of fluid directly into the small bowel during continuous infusion, which can be performed while the patient is in the CT or MR scanner. Once the small bowel is adequately distended, diagnostic enterography images can be performed. This study is not as well tolerated by patients because of the need for placement of a nasoenteric tube but enteroclysis does provide maximum small bowel distention that may be helpful in identifying subtle strictures or abnormalities hidden in poorly distended bowel.

ENTEROGRAPHY OF SMALL BOWEL DISEASES
Crohn Disease

CTE and MRE are widely used for the detection and surveillance of IBD. The performance of each technique has been shown to be similar provided the MRE is of high quality with sensitivities and specificities of greater than 80%.[5] Some institutions prefer obtaining CTE for a baseline study, given the more routinely higher image quality, and using MRE for surveillance. Other institutions that can routinely perform high-quality MRE may elect to perform MRE as the baseline study, especially in younger patients. MRE is preferred in follow-up because the various pulse sequences may allow better characterization of strictures and differentiation of inflammation from fibrosis. Several imaging findings have correlated with active inflammation, including wall thickening with mural edema, mural hyperenhancement, restricted diffusion, and engorged vasa recta (Comb sign) (**Fig. 2**). The presence of wall thickening without mural edema or hyperenhancement, upstream dilatation, and delayed enhancement suggests fibrosis.[6] However, frequently, active inflammation and fibrosis coexist.

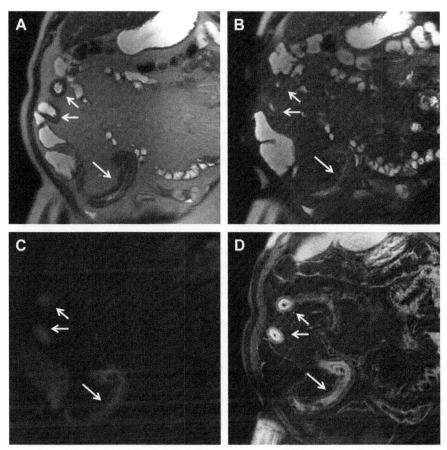

Fig. 2. MRE showing changes consistent with active inflammation in Crohn ileitis (*arrows*), including bowel wall thickening (*A*), mural edema (high T2 signal) on fat-suppressed T2-weighted images (*B*), restricted diffusion on diffusion-weighted images (*C*), and bowel wall hyperenhancement and increased vascularity following intravenous contrast (*D*).

The Society of Abdominal Radiology Disease focus panel on Crohn disease is in the process of developing standardized reporting and nomenclature in collaboration and with input from representatives of the American Gastroenterology Association's Imaging and Advanced Technology section, European Society of Gastrointestinal and Abdominal Radiology, the Society for Surgery of the Alimentary Tract, American Society of Colon and Rectal Surgeons, and North American Society for Pediatric Gastroenterology, Hepatology and Nutrition. These guidelines should be published within the next year and should result in improvements in patient care and comparison of reported research.

Cross-sectional enterography is complementary to endoscopy in the evaluation of Crohn disease. In a study, CTE detected active small bowel inflammation in more than 50% of subjects with a normal mucosa at ileoscopy due to either intramural inflammation or proximal disease out of the reach of ileoscopy.[7] Enterography has also been shown to change management in more than 50% of cases, and can find unsuspected penetrating or structuring disease, a contraindication for capsule endoscopy.[8]

There is increasing acceptance that patient symptoms do not correlate with disease activity. Therefore, there is great interest in developing and implementing imaging-based scoring systems to allow better quantification of disease activity in research trials and clinical practice. Several image-based scoring systems that vary in complexity have been derived and validated in comparison with clinical or endoscopic parameters.[9–13] Currently, there is no agreement on an accepted scoring system. These scoring systems will need further validation and improvements in analytical methods to more easily implement in clinical practice.

There are increasing data showing the utility of imaging in guiding treatment and predicting outcomes.[14] Enterography techniques can demonstrate mural inflammation that persists despite mucosal healing on endoscopy. Further studies are necessary to determine the significance of residual inflammation versus complete resolution of mural inflammation on long-term outcomes.

Gastrointestinal Bleeding

Because of the characteristics and advantages previously listed, CT is well suited for the evaluation of overt and occult lower gastrointestinal (GI) bleeding. In patients who present with overt GI bleeding, a multiphase CT angiography (CTA) can be performed quickly while the patient is actively bleeding without the need for oral contrast. CT can detect bleeding rates of 0.3 mL/min compared with 0.5 to 1.0 mL/min for angiography and 0.2 mL/min for technetium 99m (^{99m}Tc)-tagged red blood cell (TRBC) scintigraphy. In a meta-analysis, CTA had a pooled sensitivity of 89% and specificity of 85% for detecting active bleeding. It can accurately localize the site of bleeding, allowing more appropriate triaging of patients to colonoscopy, deep enteroscopy, or angiography (**Fig. 3**).[15] If the CT is negative, some clinicians have recommended watchful waiting.

In patients with occult GI bleeding a more thorough examination of the small bowel is indicated, using enterography technique as the goal is to identify the specific cause of slower or intermittent bleeding, and not the site of active extravasation as in overt bleeding. CTE has been shown to be complementary to capsule endoscopy and is superior to capsule endoscopy for detecting small bowel masses.[16,17] CTE may also identify inflammation or vascular abnormalities that may be missed on capsule endoscopy.[16] The decision to begin the small bowel evaluation with capsule endoscopy or

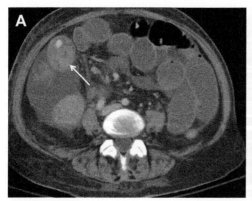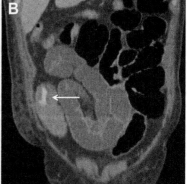

Fig. 3. Patient presenting with overt small bowel, lower GI, bleeding. Area of active bleeding is identified in the small bowel (*arrows*) on axial (*A*) and coronal (*B*) views obviating colonoscopy.

CTE will be site-dependent. However, if either technique does not identify an absolute cause for the bleeding, the alternate test should be performed. CTE should be considered as the initial test for those patients at risk for capsule retention.[18]

There are several causes responsible for small bowel bleeding. As CTE is being more widely used, knowledge is being gained about some of the subtle or unique imaging appearances of some of these diseases. A few of these abnormalities are reviewed, including vascular lesions, carcinoid tumors, and nonsteroidal antiinflammatory drug (NSAID) diaphragms.

Vascular Lesions

The imaging appearances of vascular lesions on CT have been correlated with capsule endoscopy, deep enteroscopy, and angiography.[19] CTE may allow characterization of vascular lesions based on their temporal enhancement characteristics (**Fig. 4**). High-flow lesions such as Dieulafoy lesions or arteriovenous malformations (AVMs) are usually best seen on early arterial phases and an early draining vein may be identified with AVMs (**Fig. 5**). Angioectasias appear as enlarged terminal ends of the intramural vessels and are best seen on enteric phase images with maximum intensity projection reformatted images (**Fig. 6**). Venous lesions include angiomas that show slow progressive filling and varices that appear as serpiginous intramural vessels.

Carcinoid

Carcinoid is increasing in incidence and now is the most common primary small bowel neoplasm. They may be multifocal in up to 25% of patients. With the more widespread utilization of CTE these tumors are being detected at a smaller size. These small tumors may appear as a small hyperenhancing mass in the wall of the bowel; protrude into the lumen, giving a polypoid appearance; or have a flat plaque-like appearance with retraction of the underlying wall (**Fig. 7**).

Nonsteroidal Antiinflammatory Drug Enteropathy

Short focal diaphragms can develop with NSAID enteropathy. These patients may present with small bowel bleeding and may have intermittent episodes of small bowel obstruction. The diaphragms may be subtle and often overlooked as contractions, especially when there is no significant inflammation or the bowel is poorly distended.

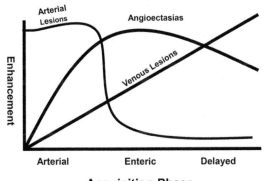

Acquisition Phase

Fig. 4. Temporal enhancement pattern of vascular lesions on CTE. (*From* Huprich JE, Barlow JM, Hansel SL, et al. Multiphase CT enterography evaluation of small-bowel vascular lesions. AJR Am J Roentgenol 2013;201(1):67; with permission.)

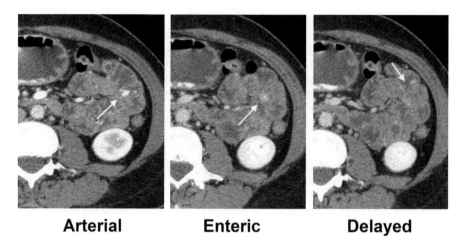

Arterial   Enteric   Delayed

Fig. 5. Actively bleeding Dieulafoy lesion (*arrows*) seen on multiphase CTE. Note the intense early enhancement on the arterial phase (*A*) that fades on the portal venous (*B*) and delayed phases (*C*). (*From* Soto JA, Park SH, Fletcher JG, et al. Gastrointestinal hemorrhage: evaluation with MDCT. Abdom Imaging 2015;40:993–1009; with permission.)

The characteristic appearance is that of multiple, adjacent, short circumferential strictures in the ileum with wall thickening, luminal narrowing, and hyperenhancement related to inflammation (**Fig. 8**). It may be difficult to differentiate these strictures from Crohn disease.

CATHETER ANGIOGRAPHY

Most traditional indications for catheter angiography in small bowel disease, evaluation of acute mesenteric ischemia, mesenteric vascular insufficiency, and chronic GI

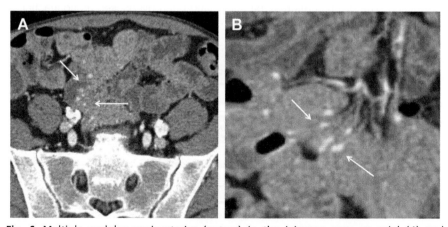

Fig. 6. Multiple nodular angioectasias (*arrows*) in the jejunum seen on axial (*A*) and maximum intensity projection reformatted (*B*) images at CTE. (*From* Huprich JE, Fletcher JG, Fidler JL, et al. Prospective blinded comparison of wireless capsule endoscopy and multiphase CT enterography in obscure gastrointestinal bleeding. Radiology 2011;260(3):744–51; with permission.)

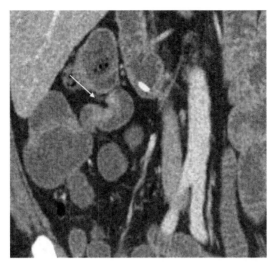

Fig. 7. Carcinoid tumor (*arrow*) with a flat morphology and underlying puckering of the bowel wall.

bleeding have been largely replaced by CTE and CTA. Catheter angiography is now used as a problem-solving modality and as part of catheter-directed interventions. Indications include the work-up of vascular disease such as vasculitis, work-up of patients with chronic GI hemorrhage, treatment of acute GI hemorrhage, guidance for surgical resection of small bowel disease, and the evaluation of the mesenteric venous system.

Vascular Disease

The evaluation of patients with either acute or chronic mesenteric ischemia now includes CTA. The use of catheter angiography is limited to patients in whom an intervention (angioplasty or arterial stent placement) is contemplated. Diagnostic angiography may be helpful when the diagnosis of vasculitis such a polyarteritis nodosa is considered. The diagnostic findings are microaneurysms involving small-to-medium sized arteries. These microaneurysms are below the threshold for detection with CT but are easily seen with catheter angiography (**Fig. 9**).

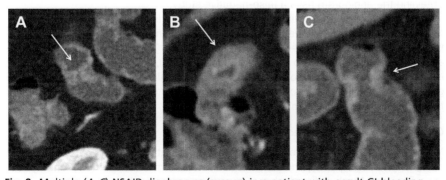

Fig. 8. Multiple (*A–C*) NSAID diaphragms (*arrows*) in a patient with occult GI bleeding.

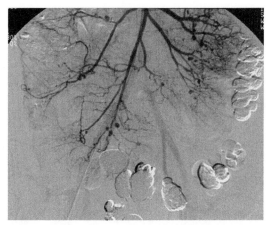

Fig. 9. Superior mesenteric angiogram demonstrating microaneurysms of multiple small arteries diagnostic of a necrotizing vasculitis such as polyarteritis nodosa.

Acute Gastrointestinal Hemorrhage

The role for catheter angiography in the patient with acute GI bleeding is to first localize the site of hemorrhage and then treat the bleeding, most commonly with selective embolization. In the past, the catheter-directed therapy for small bowel bleeding was intra-arterial vasopressin infusion. Developments in catheter and guidewire technology allowing simple subselective catheterization for embolotherapy, and the complications and failures of vasopressin infusion, render this of only historical interest.

Despite the relatively poor collateral arterial supply to the small bowel compared with the duodenum, if the embolization is carried out distally enough, the risk of bowel perforation or stricture is very low. The challenge with angiography for small bowel bleeding is timing. To treat small bowel bleeding, the bleeding itself must be seen and this requires bleeding at a rate of about 1.0 mL/min or greater because the lesion responsible for the bleeding is usually not identified. Unfortunately, bright red blood per rectum does not necessarily mean the patient is bleeding, just that they have bled. The optimal time for angiography is either immediately after a tagged red cell scan has turned positive, immediately after a positive CT scan showing active bleeding, or when there is bright red blood per rectum with ongoing hemodynamic instability. Because small bowel bleeding is frequently intermittent, any delay in obtaining the angiogram risks a false-negative study.

The basic principle in treating small bowel bleeding is to perform superior mesenteric angiography, identify the bleeding site, and advance a microcatheter as selectively as possible in the artery feeding the bleeding. The diagnostic finding is the extravasation of contrast into the bowel lumen (**Fig. 10**). The choice of embolic agent is up to the operator. Microcoils, Ivalon (polyvinyl alcohol), Gelfoam (absorbable gelatin sponge), and cyanoacrylate glue have all been described. The key is to limit to amount of bowel in the embolization zone (**Fig. 11**).

Chronic Gastrointestinal Bleeding

Many of the lesions responsible for chronic or recurrent GI bleeding can be detected by catheter angiography, including vascular malformations, tumors, aneurysms, vasculitis, and Meckel diverticulum. Other than vasculitis, these are currently best

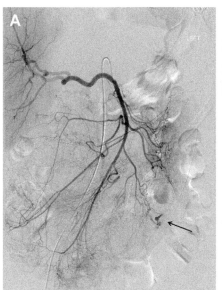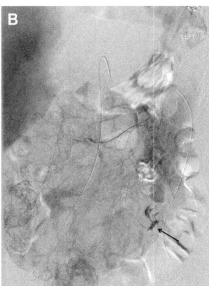

Fig. 10. Overt small bowel bleeding. Early (*A*) and late (*B*) images from an superior mesenteric artery (SMA) arteriogram. Note the contrast extravasation into the small bowel (*arrows*) that persists on the late images.

imaged with CT. Small vascular malformations may be difficult to identify at surgery, and angiography may be helpful. A microcatheter can be placed into the malformation's feeding artery, and the patient transported to surgery. After the abdomen is opened, methylene blue is slowly injected into the feeding artery, identifying the segment of bowel encompassing the vascular malformation (**Fig. 12**). Although these lesions may be treated with embolotherapy, the recurrence rate is significant, so surgical resection is preferred if a patient's clinical condition permits.

An evolving role for angiography is the treatment of bleeding metastases to the GI tract.[20] Although this therapy is most applicable to the stomach and duodenum, in selected patients, tumors metastatic to the small bowel may be treated with selective embolization (**Fig. 13**).

Mesenteric Venous System

Stenosis or occlusion of the superior mesenteric vein (SMV) can lead to bowel edema and pain, ascites and GI bleeding. Common causes include tumor encasement, complications of surgery, and pancreatitis. The lesions are detected by cross-sectional imaging, which is used for procedural planning. The portal system can be accessed from either the transhepatic or trans-splenic approach to allow attempted recanalization and stenting of the occluded or stenotic segment.[21] The ideal patient has a short segment lesion of the main trunk of the SMV (**Fig. 14**), although more complex lesions can be treated in selected cases (**Fig. 15**).

EMERGING NUCLEAR MEDICINE AND PET TECHNIQUES

Interesting developments have occurred in radionuclide small intestine imaging due to emergence of hybrid imaging modalities such as single-photon emission CT-CT (SPECT/CT), PET/CT, and PET/MRI. The following section updates referring providers

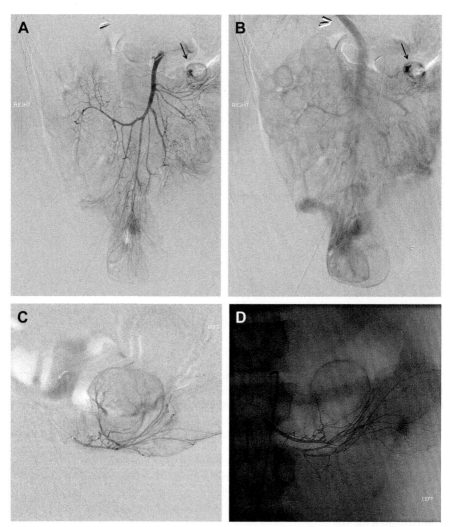

Fig. 11. Overt bleeding with Gelfoam embolization. Superior mesenteric angiogram shows extravasation of contrast (*arrows*) into the proximal jejunum (*A*) that persists into the portal venous phase (*B*). Selective injection of the first jejunal artery (*C*) defines the branch responsible for the hemorrhage. Follow-up injection of the first jejunal artery after subselective embolization of the bleeding branch with small pieces of Gelfoam confirms control of the bleeding, with preservation of as much jejunal arterial supply as possible (*D*).

on the background and salient features of the investigations that have been influenced by these developments.

Tagged Red Blood Cell Study for Gastrointestinal Bleeding of Small Bowel Origin

Red blood cell (RBC) scintigraphy, also TRBC scan, has been used for detection and localization of the source of bleeding in patients with acute GI bleeding. It involves tagging the circulating blood with the radionuclide ^{99m}Tc. The test is based on the principle of detection of extravasated tagged blood at the bleeding site within the GI tract using a gamma camera. Delayed imaging with the same injection of TRBC can be

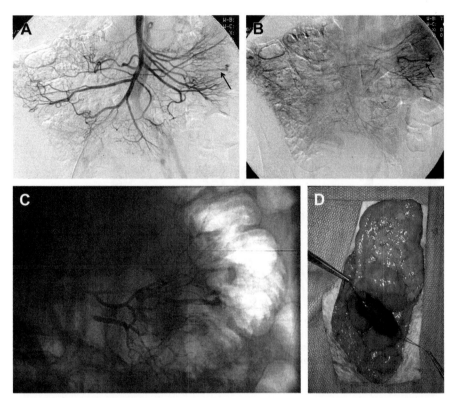

Fig. 12. Vascular malformation with preoperative mapping. Arterial (*A*) and early venous (*B*) superior mesenteric angiograms demonstrating an early draining vein from a tiny, small bowel vascular malformation (*arrows*). A microcatheter was placed into the feeding artery (*C*) and, in the operating room, methylene blue was slowly injected, marking the segment of bowel to be resected (*D*).

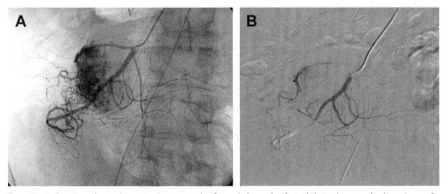

Fig. 13. Selective ileocolic arteriograms before (*A*) and after (*B*) Ivalon embolization of a small bowel metastasis from renal cell carcinoma to the distal ilium and cecum.

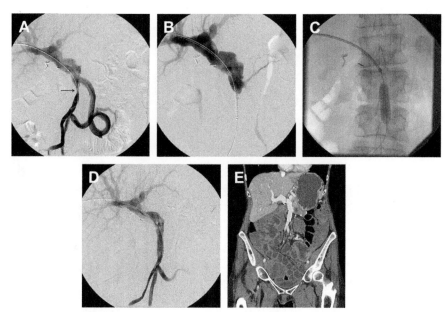

Fig. 14. A 65-year-old woman presents with small bowel varices following a Whipple procedure. Transhepatic venogram (*A*) shows a tight stenosis (*arrow*) of the SMV with varices. This was treated with a balloon expandable stent (*B, C*) with good result (*D*). CT obtained 39 months after stent placement show a widely patent SMV stent with persistent resolution of her varices (*E*).

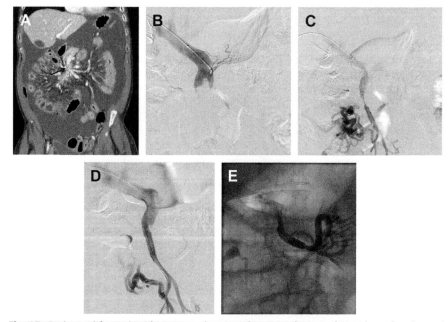

Fig. 15. Patient with carcinoid tumor and ascites due to occlusion of SMV branches (*arrow*) (*A*). Portal venogram shows 2 large branch occlusions (*B*). Both were crossed, dilated, and stented open (*C–E*). Ascites has resolved at 5-month follow-up.

performed if the bleeding is not identified in the initial hour of dynamic imaging. However, the utility of delayed imaging is uncertain, given that active bleeding must be detected dynamically to confidently identify an anatomic source. In general, planar TRBC scintigraphy is sensitive for detection of acute bleeding.[22] Highest diagnostic yield is obtained if the test is performed when the patient has symptoms suggestive of active bleeding. Although animal studies suggest that scintigraphy can detect as low as 0.1 mL/min bleed rate, it is thought that an in vitro bleed rate 2 to 3 times this level would be required to detect the site of bleed with this study. However, the accuracy of TRBC scan for localization of bleeding source is debatable due to the limited spatial resolution (anatomic definition) of traditional planar mode.[22–24] This is especially true in patients with complex intra-abdominal anatomy due to multiple prior surgeries. Determination of whether the bleeding is from the small or large intestine can also be a challenge. Pooling of the radiotracer in normal structures can sometimes lead to false-positive errors. These factors contribute to uncertainty regarding the appropriate use of this test in the management of patients with acute GI bleeding.

Recently, SPECT/CT has been used to address some limitations of planar bleeding scan.[25–27] SPECT/CT is a hybrid imaging modality that consists of 2 hardwired juxtaposed machines, a gamma camera, and a multidetector CT with a common patient bed and a single computer console. It involves sequential volumetric scintigraphic acquisition-reconstruction and a low-radiation dose, free-breathing CT scan without a change in patient position. The CT data are used for attenuation correction and anatomic colocalization of scintigraphic data. In addition, the technique entails automated coregistration of cross-sectional SPECT and CT images, which allows intuitive multiplanar display of radiotracer distribution superimposed on anatomy. Recent studies have demonstrated the feasibility of performing SPECT/CT immediately after planar TRBC study in subjects with acute GI bleeding. For instance, Goenka and colleagues[25] reviewed their experience with 29 subjects who had a concurrent hybrid SPECT/CT for evaluating equivocal TRBC activity on planar scintigraphy. Average additional time required for SPECT/CT was 20 minutes (range: 13–31). In 9 subjects with apparently positive results on planar study, SPECT/CT demonstrated that scintigraphic activity was actually due to non-GI causes (**Fig. 16**). In the remaining subjects, the SPECT/CT localized scintigraphic TRBC activity to within the GI tract. The source of bleeding thus identified on SPECT/CT was found concordant with the source confirmed through subsequent diagnostic and therapeutic interventions (**Fig. 17**). Thus, additional SPECT/CT fusion imaging correctly localized GI bleeding source with minimal time and radiation penalty. It also reduced ambiguities in interpretation of planar scintigraphy by identifying the confounding, non-GI sources of TRBC activity owing to optimal demonstration of regional anatomy. Likewise, Kotani and colleagues[28] have demonstrated incremental diagnostic yield for detection of acute GI bleeding and for identifying the source of bleeding by combining hybrid SPECT/CT with planar scintigraphy with another commonly used radiotracer: ^{99m}Tc-human serum albumin- diethylenetriamine-pentaacetic acid (DTPA). In anecdotal reports, SPECT/CT has also facilitated accurate identification of Meckel diverticulum as the source of abdominal pain and GI bleeding.[29]

Hybrid SPECT/CT clearly has the potential to improve the clinical utility of planar RBC scintigraphy in acute GI bleeding and represents an important advance. Certain limitations, however, merit consideration. First, availability is not universal and can be an issue especially in the after-hours when the planar TRBC study is often performed. Second, rapid antegrade or retrograde movement of the extravasated luminal tracer away from the site of bleeding due to increased peristalsis can be a potential confounder. However, this has not been observed in previously referenced studies.

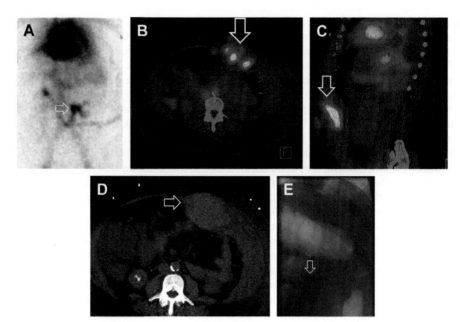

Fig. 16. Rectus sheath hematoma mimicking GI bleed on planar RBC scintigraphy. A 60-year-old man patient with end-stage liver disease, portal hypertension, large-volume ascites, and acute drop in hemoglobin and hematocrit was evaluated with planar RBC scintigraphy to assess for acute GI bleed. Planar image demonstrated an ambiguous focus of activity in the left lower quadrant (*arrow* in *A*) that increased in intensity over time and it was not clear whether this was small or large bowel. SPECT/CT demonstrated that the focus was actually centered in the left rectus sheath (*arrows* in *B* and *C*). Noncontrast CT confirmed a rectus sheath hematoma (*arrow* in *D*). On invasive angiogram, this was found to be due to an actively bleeding pseudoaneurysm from the inferior epigastric artery (*arrow* in *E*), which was likely due to repeated paracentesis on the floor.

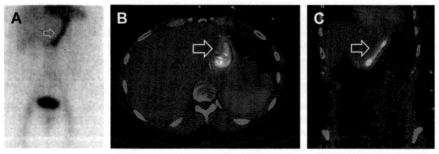

Fig. 17. Overt bleeding within excluded stomach. A 42-year old man with remote history of Roux-en-Y gastric bypass (RYGB) presented with hematemesis. Endoscopy and visceral angiography were negative. Planar RBC scintigraphy demonstrated tracer localization in the stomach (*arrow* in *A*) that increased in intensity over time but the interpretation was confounded in the setting of prior RYGB and negative endoscopy. SPECT/CT localized the tracer to the excluded stomach (*arrows* in *B* and *C*). Exploratory laparotomy confirmed that this was due to a bleeding ulcer in the excluded stomach, which escaped detection on endoscopy of the gastric pouch.

Moreover, the technique has not yet been validated in large, prospective studies and the patient population most likely to benefit from it has not been defined. Finally, direct comparison with other cross-sectional imaging modalities such as CT has not been done and improvements in outcomes due to the use of hybrid SPECT/CT has not been investigated.

Inflammatory Bowel Disease

Recent developments in hybrid imaging modalities using the radiotracer 2-[18F] fluoro-2-deoxy-D-glucose (FDG) have demonstrated new opportunities for molecular imaging of IBD. FDG is a relatively nonspecific radiotracer. In addition to neoplasms, it is also taken up by inflammatory cells. Therefore, FDG PET/CT and FDG PET/MR have been evaluated as noninvasive investigations for assessment of active inflammation in patients with IBD in several small studies.

On PET/CT, inflamed bowel segments tend to show FDG uptake higher than the subadjacent uninvolved bowel, as well as higher than the FDG uptake in normal liver parenchyma. Several small studies have shown that FDG PET/CT can assess the extent, location, and disease activity in patients with suspected as well as known IBD[30–32] In general, PET/CT-identified segments of active inflammation correlate well with the standard investigations such as CTE or MRE and endoscopy. A pooled analysis of 7 studies has demonstrated 85% sensitivity and 87% specificity in assessing IBD on a per-segment analysis and 93.3% area under the receiver operating characteristic (ROC) curve for FDG PET and PET/CT.[33] Absence of FDG uptake in morphologically abnormal intestinal segments on CTE has been shown to be associated with failure of medical therapy.[30] Limited data also show that FDG PET/CT-identified bowel inflammation decreases with medical treatment and correlates with symptom improvement.[34]

However, accurate assessment of complications on FDG PET/CT is not feasible due to limited anatomic resolution and lack of bowel distension. On PET alone, differentiation of physiologic bowel FDG uptake from pathologic uptake can be a challenge. Risks of radiation exposure resulting from longitudinal surveillance imaging are also a real concern. The CT component of PET/CT is a low-dose, free-breathing acquisition. Therefore, it does not allow accurate anatomic evaluation of those bowel segments that demonstrate increased FDG uptake. Assessment can also be confounded by misregistration artifacts due to sequential acquisition of PET and CT. It has been suggested that the CT component of the PET/CT may be improved through the use of PET/CT enteroclysis.[35] Although technically feasible, this is often not practical. Improvements in technique that facilitate faster data acquisition at reduced radiation dose and development of radiotracers that are specific for inflamed segments may facilitate wider clinical use of PET/CT in patients with IBD.

One critical challenge in patients with Crohn disease is differentiation of inflammatory from fibrotic strictures. None of the currently available noninvasive imaging modalities, including FDG PET/CT, allow this distinction with high accuracy.[36,37] Recently, a new hybrid molecular imaging modality, PET/MRI, has shown promise in making this distinction. A truly integrated PET/MRI combines PET detectors and MRI in a single gantry to enable simultaneous acquisition of PET and MR data, resulting in excellent temporal and spatial coregistration. This offers the opportunity for simultaneous assessment of complementary anatomic, functional, and metabolic information.

PET/MR evaluation of small bowel has been shown to be technically feasible with reasonable coregistration of small intestine segments on fused PET/MRI images.[38] Quantitative biomarkers from FDG PET/MR combined with MRE have shown promise in distinguishing inflammatory from purely fibrotic strictures in patients with CD.[39] In general, fibrotic strictures tended to show lower signal intensity on T2-weighted images and apparent diffusion coefficient (ADC) value on diffusion-weighted imaging sequences of MRE, and lower maximum standardized uptake value (SUVmax) on PET/MR. A hybrid biomarker, namely product of SUVmax (derived from PET/MR) and ADC (derived from MRE), performed better than markers from either modality alone, although the trend was not statistically significant. Nevertheless, this distinguishing ability derived from quantitative biomarkers when combined with other information such as disease activity, and complications obtained from the MRE component, show the potential of PET/MRE as a 1-stop-shop imaging study for Crohn disease. This advance represents an exciting opportunity. If validated, it has the potential to become the standard-of-care in differentiating inflammatory from fibrotic strictures in patients with Crohn disease. Moreover, the technique may offer a novel imaging option for response assessment of the antifibrotic agents that are in various stages of development.[39–41]

However, PET/MRI is currently an investigational tool and is available only at a few academic centers. There are no standardized PET/MR protocols in the literature for evaluation of small bowel, which is a reflection of the novelty of this modality. Although it offers several advantages compared with PET/CT, such as reduced radiation, superior soft tissue contrast resolution, and a wide range of data acquisition, its workflow is a major challenge and several technical aspects need to be addressed. PET/MRI also needs to be compared directly with CTE and MRE, which are part of the current standard-of-care for IBD. Validation of the technique in prospective studies and the most appropriate patient population that will benefit from its application also need to be defined.

In summary, IBD is a novel indication for FDG PET studies. Initial studies with hybrid imaging modalities such as PET/CT and PET/MR have shown promising results. PET is likely to find application in selected patient populations for answering specific clinical questions.

REFERENCES

1. Baker ME, Hara AK, Platt JF, et al. CT enterography for Crohn's disease: optimal technique and imaging issues. Abdom Imaging 2015;40(5):938–52.
2. Gandhi NS, Baker ME, Goenka AH, et al. Diagnostic accuracy of CT enterography for active inflammatory terminal ileal Crohn disease: comparison of full-dose and half-dose images reconstructed with FBP and half-dose images with SAFIRE. Radiology 2016;280(2):436–45.
3. Lee SJ, Park SH, Kim AY, et al. A prospective comparison of standard-dose CT enterography and 50% reduced-dose CT enterography with and without noise reduction for evaluating Crohn disease. AJR Am J Roentgenol 2011;197(1):50–7.
4. Kolbe AB, Fletcher JG, Froemming AT, et al. Evaluation of Patient Tolerance and Small-Bowel Distention With a New Small-Bowel Distending Agent for Enterography. AJR Am J Roentgenol 2016;206(5):994–1002.
5. Qiu Y, Mao R, Chen BL, et al. Systematic review with meta-analysis: magnetic resonance enterography vs. computed tomography enterography for evaluating disease activity in small bowel Crohn's disease. Aliment Pharmacol Ther 2014; 40(2):134–46.
6. Rimola J, Planell N, Rodriguez S, et al. Characterization of inflammation and fibrosis in Crohn's disease lesions by magnetic resonance imaging. Am J Gastroenterol 2015;110(3):432–40.

7. Samuel S, Bruining DH, Loftus EV Jr, et al. Endoscopic skipping of the distal ter-minal ileum in Crohn's disease can lead to negative results from ileocolonoscopy. Clin Gastroenterol Hepatol 2012;10(11):1253–9.

8. Bruining DH, Siddiki HA, Fletcher JG, et al. Benefit of computed tomography en-terography in Crohn's disease: effects on patient management and physician level of confidence. Inflamm Bowel Dis 2012;18(2):219–25.

9. Makanyanga JC, Pendse D, Dikaios N, et al. Evaluation of Crohn's disease activ-ity: initial validation of a magnetic resonance enterography global score (MEGS) against faecal calprotectin. Eur Radiol 2014;24(2):277–87.

10. Oussalah A, Laurent V, Bruot O, et al. Diffusion-weighted magnetic resonance without bowel preparation for detecting colonic inflammation in inflammatory bowel disease. Gut 2010;59(8):1056–65.

11. Pariente B, Mary JY, Danese S, et al. Development of the Lemann index to assess digestive tract damage in patients with Crohn's disease. Gastroenterology 2015; 148(1):52–63.e3.

12. Rimola J, Rodriguez S, Garcia-Bosch O, et al. Magnetic resonance for assess-ment of disease activity and severity in ileocolonic Crohn's disease. Gut 2009; 58(8):1113–20.

13. Steward MJ, Punwani S, Proctor I, et al. Non-perforating small bowel Crohn's dis-ease assessed by MRI enterography: derivation and histopathological validation of an MR-based activity index. Eur J Radiol Sep 2012;81(9):2080–8.

14. Deepak P, Fletcher JG, Fidler JL, et al. Radiological response is associated with better long-term outcomes and is a potential treatment target in patients with small bowel Crohn's disease. Am J Gastroenterol 2016;111(7):997–1006.

15. Wu LM, Xu JR, Yin Y, et al. Usefulness of CT angiography in diagnosing acute gastrointestinal bleeding: a meta-analysis. World J Gastroenterol 2010;16(31): 3957–63.

16. Huprich JE, Fletcher JG, Fidler JL, et al. Prospective blinded comparison of wire-less capsule endoscopy and multiphase CT enterography in obscure gastrointes-tinal bleeding. Radiology 2011;260(3):744–51.

17. Wang Z, Chen JQ, Liu JL, et al. CT enterography in obscure gastrointestinal bleeding: a systematic review and meta-analysis. J Med Imaging Radiat Oncol 2013;57(3):263–73.

18. Gerson LB, Fidler JL, Cave DR, et al. ACG clinical guideline: diagnosis and man-agement of small bowel bleeding. Am J Gastroenterol 2015;110(9):1265–87 [quiz: 1288].

19. Huprich JE, Barlow JM, Hansel SL, et al. Multiphase CT enterography evaluation of small-bowel vascular lesions. AJR Am J Roentgenol Jul 2013;201(1):65–72.

20. Tandberg DJ, Smith TP, Suhocki PV, et al. Early outcomes of empiric embolization of tumor-related gastrointestinal hemorrhage in patients with advanced malig-nancy. J Vasc Interv Radiol 2012;23(11):1445–52.

21. Woodrum DA, Bjarnason H, Andrews JC. Portal vein venoplasty and stent place-ment in the nontransplant population. J Vasc Interv Radiol 2009;20(5):593–9.

22. Allen TW, Tulchinsky M. Nuclear medicine tests for acute gastrointestinal condi-tions. Semin Nucl Med 2013;43(2):88–101.

23. Currie GM, Kiat H, Wheat JM. Scintigraphic evaluation of acute lower gastrointes-tinal hemorrhage: current status and future directions. J Clin Gastroenterol 2011; 45(2):92–9.

24. Dolezal J, Kopacova M. Radionuclide small intestine imaging. Gastroenterol Res Pract 2013;2013:861619.

25. Goenka AH, Shrikanthan S, Neumann DN. Localization of gastrointestinal bleeding with hybrid SPECT/CT in patients with equivocal bleeding source on a positive 99mTc-labeled RBC dynamic planar scintigraphy. Paper presented at American Roentgen Ray Society Annual Meeting. May 8, San Diego (CA), 2014.

26. Schillaci O, Spanu A, Tagliabue L, et al. SPECT/CT with a hybrid imaging system in the study of lower gastrointestinal bleeding with technetium-99m red blood cells. Q J Nucl Med Mol Imaging 2009;53(3):281–9.

27. Yamamoto Y, Nishiyama Y. SPECT/CT imaging in (9)(9)mTc-HSA-DTPA gastrointestinal bleeding scintigraphy to localize bleeding sites. Eur J Nucl Med Mol Imaging 2012;39(11):1824–5.

28. Kotani K, Kawabe J, Higashiyama S, et al. Diagnostic ability of (99m)Tc-HSA-DTPA scintigraphy in combination with SPECT/CT for gastrointestinal bleeding. Abdom Imaging 2014;39(4):677–84.

29. Turgeon DK, Brenner D, Brown RK, et al. Possible role of Meckel's scan fused with SPECT CT imaging: unraveling the cause of abdominal pain and obscure-overt gastrointestinal bleeding. Case Rep Gastroenterol 2008;2(1):83–90.

30. Ahmadi A, Li Q, Muller K, et al. Diagnostic value of noninvasive combined fluorine-18 labeled fluoro-2-deoxy-D-glucose positron emission tomography and computed tomography enterography in active Crohn's disease. Inflamm Bowel Dis 2010;16(6):974–81.

31. Malham M, Hess S, Nielsen RG, et al. PET/CT in the diagnosis of inflammatory bowel disease in pediatric patients: a review. Am J Nucl Med Mol Imaging 2014;4(3):225–30.

32. Perlman SB, Hall BS, Reichelderfer M. PET/CT imaging of inflammatory bowel disease. Semin Nucl Med 2013;43(6):420–6.

33. Treglia G, Quartuccio N, Sadeghi R, et al. Diagnostic performance of Fluorine-18-Fluorodeoxyglucose positron emission tomography in patients with chronic inflammatory bowel disease: a systematic review and a meta-analysis. J Crohns Colitis 2013;7(5):345–54.

34. Spier BJ, Perlman SB, Jaskowiak CJ, et al. PET/CT in the evaluation of inflammatory bowel disease: studies in patients before and after treatment. Mol Imaging Biol 2010;12(1):85–8.

35. Das CJ, Makharia G, Kumar R, et al. PET-CT enteroclysis: a new technique for evaluation of inflammatory diseases of the intestine. Eur J Nucl Med Mol Imaging 2007;34(12):2106–14.

36. Jacene HA, Ginsburg P, Kwon J, et al. Prediction of the need for surgical intervention in obstructive Crohn's disease by 18F-FDG PET/CT. J Nucl Med 2009;50(11):1751–9.

37. Lenze F, Wessling J, Bremer J, et al. Detection and differentiation of inflammatory versus fibromatous Crohn's disease strictures: prospective comparison of 18F-FDG-PET/CT, MR-enteroclysis, and transabdominal ultrasound versus endoscopic/histologic evaluation. Inflamm Bowel Dis 2012;18(12):2252–60.

38. Beiderwellen K, Kinner S, Gomez B, et al. Hybrid imaging of the bowel using PET/MR enterography: Feasibility and first results. Eur J Radiol 2016;85(2):414–21.

39. Catalano OA, Gee MS, Nicolai E, et al. Evaluation of Quantitative PET/MR Enterography Biomarkers for Discrimination of Inflammatory Strictures from Fibrotic Strictures in Crohn Disease. Radiology 2016;278(3):792–800.

40. Latella G, Sferra R, Speca S, et al. Can we prevent, reduce or reverse intestinal fibrosis in IBD? Eur Rev Med Pharmacol Sci 2013;17(10):1283–304.

41. Rieder F, Fiocchi C. Intestinal fibrosis in IBD–a dynamic, multifactorial process. Nat Rev Gastroenterol Hepatol 2009;6(4):228–35.

Intraoperative Enteroscopy
Is There Still a Role?

Thibault Voron, MD[a,b], Gabriel Rahmi, MD, PhD[b,c],
Stephane Bonnet, MD[d], Georgia Malamut, MD, PhD[b,c],
Philippe Wind, MD[e,f], Christophe Cellier, MD, PhD[b,c],
Anne Berger, MD[a,b], Richard Douard, MD, PhD[a,b,*]

KEYWORDS

- Intraoperative enteroscopy • Obscure gastrointestinal bleeding • Laparotomy
- Digestive surgery • Small bowel

KEY POINTS

- Vascular lesions are the major cause of obscure gastrointestinal bleeding. Their treatment is mainly endoscopic, radiologic, medical, and less and less surgical. IOE is responsible for endoscopy-induced traumatic lesions that are difficult to distinguish from true vascular lesions.
- The development of deep enteroscopy and video-capsule endoscopy has reduced the indications for diagnostic intraoperative enteroscopy (IOE) which remains still indicated in rare cases when preoperative noninvasive small bowel exploration techniques are not available, or when there are preoperative conflicting results.
- The negative predictive value of the noninvasive small bowel exploration is so high that it is recommended to repeat conventional upper and lower endoscopy in cases of negative video-capsule endoscopy and/or overtube-assisted endoscopy explorations.

Continued

The authors have nothing to disclose.
[a] Department of General and Digestive Surgery, Georges Pompidou European AP-HP University Hospital, 20-40 rue Leblanc, 75908 Paris Cedex 15, France; [b] Paris Descartes Faculty of Medicine, 15, rue de l'Ecole de Médecine, Paris 75006, France; [c] Department of Gastroenterology and Endoscopy, Georges Pompidou European AP-HP University Hospital, 20-40, rue Leblanc, 75908 Paris Cedex 15, France; [d] Department of Digestive Surgery, Percy University Military Hospital, 101 Avenue Henri Barbusse, Clamart 92140, France; [e] Department of Digestive Surgery, Avicenne AP-HP University Hospital, 125 Rue de Stalingrad, Bobigny 93000, France; [f] UFR SMBH, Paris-Nord University, 74, rue Marcel Cachin, 93017 Bobigny cedex, France
* Corresponding author. Service de Chirurgie Générale et Digestive, Hôpital européen Georges Pompidou, 20-40, rue Leblanc, Paris 75908 Cedex 15, France.
E-mail address: richard.douard@aphp.fr

Gastrointest Endoscopy Clin N Am 27 (2017) 153–170
http://dx.doi.org/10.1016/j.giec.2016.08.009
1052-5157/17/© 2016 Elsevier Inc. All rights reserved.

Continued

- When preoperative small bowel explorations are negative, the probability of finding abnormality on IOE is significantly low so that it should only be performed if the clinical suspicion of finding a lesion is very high.
- Therapeutic IOE remains indicated to guide the intraoperative treatment of small bowel lesions identified by a preoperative workup that cannot be managed by angiographic embolization and/or endoscopic treatment and cannot be localized during surgical explorations (ie, no serosal visible lesion and/or no previous tattoo).

INTRODUCTION

Obscure gastrointestinal bleeding (OGIB) remains a great diagnostic challenge because bleeding can arise from the small bowel in 45% to 75% of cases. The small bowel remains a difficult part of the digestive tract to access. Video-capsule endoscopy (VCE) and deep enteroscopy have made it possible to explore the entire small bowel. Moreover, deep enteroscopy has provided the possibility of endoscopically treating most lesions responsible for bleeding. If enteroscopy failed to reach the lesion, intraoperative enteroscopy represents the last resort diagnostic technique to explore the entire small bowel. This procedure was associated with a relatively high morbidity and mortality. Thus, indications for IOE have decreased, and some investigators now consider that IOE can no more be considered a diagnostic tool but a guiding technique to manage preoperatively small bowel mucosal lesions when other techniques, including laparoscopy and laparotomy, failed to discover a bleeding lesion. There is still some debate on the indication for IOE when preoperative small bowel explorations are negative or with conflicting results. In such cases, some investigators still consider IOE the last resort diagnostic tool.[1]

The aim of the present work was to determine the remaining indications for IOE through a literature and expert opinion review. The authors successively answer the following questions: How is an intraoperative enteroscopy performed? What is the diagnostic and therapeutic yield of this procedure, and what is the bleeding recurrence rate? What is the morbidity of IOE? What is the current role for IOE in the exploration of obscure gastrointestinal (GI) bleeding?

How to Perform an Intraoperative Enteroscopy

IOE associates abdominal exploration and intraoperative enteroscopy itself. The challenging question is whether to perform IOE when abdominal exploration discovered a potential cause for GI bleeding. On one hand, abdominal exploration is a good occasion to perform a complete exploration of small bowel by an IOE. On the other hand, when a cause for GI bleeding has been potentially localized during the abdominal exploration, a subsequent negative IOE[2,3] carries the risks of morbidity due to distension of the mesentery.

Abdominal exploration is usually performed via midline laparotomy even though the laparoscopic approach has been reported in case reports and small series.[4–8] The former history of abdominal surgery has to be taken into account when an IOE is indicated. Complete adhesiolysis must first be performed carefully to avoid creating iatrogenic lesions during enteroscopy, which could be mistaken for bleeding lesions at endoscopy. A complete surgical exploration of the abdomen is mandatory to exclude macroscopic abnormalities. It includes the exploration of the stomach, duodenum, and the entire length of the large and small intestines using the transillumination technique. When macroscopic lesions are found, the surgeon has to evaluate the probability of whether these lesions are causing GI bleeding and to decide whether to perform IOE.

After the complete surgical exploration, IOE itself has to be prepared. IOE can be performed using the peroral technique, the transanal technique, one or more enterotomies, or combined techniques (**Fig. 1**; see **Table 2**). Standard enteroscopy with or without overtube might be preferred instead of use of an adult colonoscope because the enteroscope is thinner and probably less traumatic for the small bowel. CO_2 insufflation during endoscopic procedure instead of air insufflation is also recommended to avoid too much intestinal wall distension. When peroral technique is considered, the Kocher maneuver is recommended to divide the hepatoduodenal ligament and separate the head of the pancreas from the right retroperitoneum. Then, mobilization of the duodenojejunal junction, that is, division of the ligament of Treitz, has also to be performed. When the transanal approach is considered, the extended mobilization of the colon (ie, ileocecal junction, right colon, and hepatic flexure mobilization) is recommended.

The transoral approach is the least invasive procedure, but it is often difficult to reach the terminal ileum.[9–11] In these cases, another approach is needed, either an enterotomy or a transanal approach. The advantage of combining the transoral and the transanal approach when the transoral approach only does not allow access to the terminal ileum, is that performing an enterotomy during surgery can be avoided. In return, this combined approach is time consuming and could generate a large distension of the small bowel and the colon, which may lead to difficulties in closing the abdominal wall. To avoid these difficulties, an enterotomy can be conducted to explore the previously unexplored small bowel during the transoral approach.[2,12]

The systematic enterotomy approach is currently used in laparoscopically assisted IOE.[4,5,7,8] The question of whether to perform an enterotomy only for complete small bowel exploration is a rare event. In most cases, the great part of the small bowel has been explored by the peroral approach, and some lesions have been marked for further small bowel resection. These resection sites can be used as enterotomies for complete small bowel exploration. In some rare cases, when IOE by peroral approach is negative, the transanal approach could be used to avoid the risks for an enterotomy but with the problems of major intestinal and colonic distension.

The transoral approach starts by the introduction of the enteroscope in the duodenum through the pylorus under visual control and manual guidance. It is then guided by the surgeon through the third and fourth portions of duodenum until it crosses the duodenojejunal flexure.

For some investigators, it is best to perform this step of the procedure before completion of the midline laparotomy because the adhesions facilitate the passage of enteroscope through the duodenum. The critical point of this step in the procedure is then to avoid an intragastric loop, which is possible by using an overtube to prevent the endoscope from curving along the great curvature of the stomach.

When the transoral approach does not allow exploration of the last portion of the small bowel, endoscopists can combine this approach with the transanal approach or with use of intraoperative enterotomy performed by the surgeon.

Several technical refinements have been described to minimalize intraoperative contamination, such as a circular suture surrounding the bowel, the use of a sterile laparoscopic plastic sheath that is temporarily sutured to the borders of the enterotomy,[3] or the use of a laparoscopic 15-mm trocart to introduce the endoscope through the enterotomy.[13] This approach divides the small bowel into 2 shorter segments. The

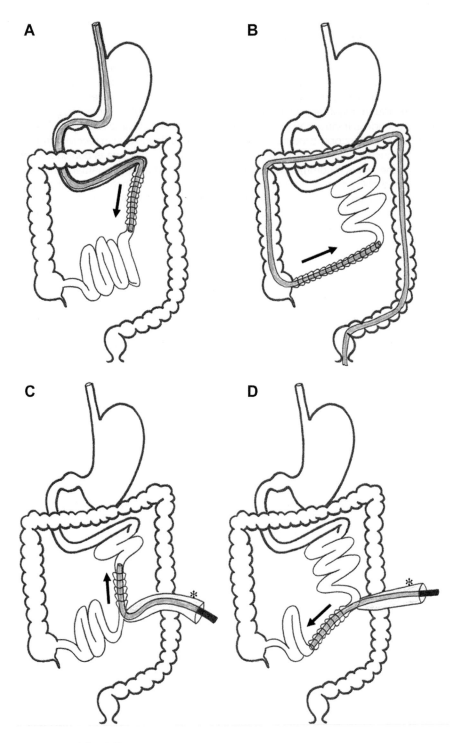

Fig. 1. View of the different approaches that may be combined to perform an intraoperative enteroscopy. (*A*) Transoral approach. (*B*) Transanal approach. (*C*) Enterotomy approach

insertion and removal of the endoscope is performed by a surgeon, with other maneuvers usually performed by an endoscopist.

During intraoperative enteroscopy, the small bowel has to be explored completely to avoid missing some lesions. For this purpose, a dual examination is performed, both internally and directly by the endoscopist through the enteroscope, but also externally by the surgeon with the transilluminated bowel. In the literature and in the authors' experience, insufflation is performed using the nonsterile air of the operating room. For optimal small bowel mucosa visualization, the "air-trapping" technique is the most suitable and consists of pinching a segment of the bowel with fingers to trap sufficient air to keep the lumen open. This technique minimizes mucosal trauma and avoids the use of traumatic clamps and excessive insufflations. Noncrushing occluding clamps can be used and positioned at the ileocecal valve and the duodenojejunal junction, but the authors do not use them due to the risks of intestinal damage. Once a segment has been examined, it is pleated over the endoscope, and the next part of the intestine segment can be examined. This procedure is repeated throughout the entire small bowel, and the surgeon manually advances the endoscope by telescoping the bowel over the tip.

Unlike a colonoscopy, it is essential that the intestinal mucosa be explored during the progression of the enteroscope and not during its withdrawal. Indeed, the progression of the enteroscope, even with the specific "air-trapping" technique described above, may cause trauma of the intestinal mucosa, which may then be considered a vascular lesion during withdrawal of the enteroscope. Lesions identified during intraoperative enteroscopy are then marked with suture stitches on the serosal surface of the small bowel to locate the sites of future segmental resection if endoscopic treatment is unsuitable. Then, careful exsufflation is performed.

Complete enteroscopy depends on several factors, such as the experience of the team or surgical constraints. However, the feasibility rate of complete enteroscopy has been reported to range from 57% to 100%.[1,10,11,14–16]

Diagnostic and Therapeutic Yield of Intraoperative Enteroscopy in the Management of Obscure Gastrointestinal Bleeding

The literature search identified 16 publications in which intraoperative enteroscopy was assessed.[1–3,9–11,14–23] In, total, 468 patients who underwent intraoperative enteroscopy were included. According to the previously published data (see **Table 2**), a site-specific source of bleeding was detected in 371 patients (79.27%), confirming that the source of bleeding in OGIB is often located in the small bowel. The predominant lesions responsible for OGIB and identified by IOE were vascular lesions, which represented 61% (n = 227) of findings, as described previously.[24,25] The remaining lesion types were as follows: benign ulcers in 19% (n = 70), tumors in 10% (n = 36), and diverticula in 4.0% (n = 15).

---

to explore the proximal small bowel, for example, when an additional enterotomy is performed to complete a transanal approach. (*D*) Enterotomy approach to explore the distal small bowel, for example, when an additional enterotomy is performed to complete a transoral approach. When an exclusive enterotomy approach is used, (*C*) and (*D*) are combined. (*Asterisk*) The endoscope is introduced in a mid-small bowel enterotomy through a sterile laparoscopic plastic sheath temporarily sutured to the borders of the enterotomy. The *black arrow* represents the direction of endoscope insertion. (*From* Bonnet S, Douard R, Malamut G, et al. Intraoperative enteroscopy in the management of obscure gastrointestinal bleeding. Dig Liver Dis 2013;45:281; with permission.)

Endoscopic or histologic data that distinguished the different types of vascular lesions (ie, angiodysplasias, arteriovenous malformation) were lacking in the published studies. In the case of small bowel resection, histologic confirmation of vascular lesions cannot be regularly obtained. Diagnosis is then usually endoscopic and, therefore, uncertain. Final pathologic examination confirmed the vascular lesions visualized during IOE in 62% to 100% of cases.[10,14,18] The complete list of intraoperative findings is summarized in **Table 1**.

Table 1
Intraoperative endoscopic small bowel findings of 464 patients from 16 series

Intraoperative Endoscopic Findings	No. of Patients
Vascular lesions (n = 227)	
Small bowel angiodysplasia	161
Arteriovenous malformations	41
Colonic angiodysplasia	9
Arteriovenous malformations and associated ulcers	3
Jejunal varices	3
Hemangioma	3
Rendu-Osler-Weber disease	2
Small bowel Dieulafoy lesion	3
Colonic Dieulafoy lesion	1
Jejunal hamartoma	1
Benign ulcers (n = 70)	
Small bowel ulcers (including Crohn ulcerations)	70
Tumors (n = 36)	
Small bowel tumor	25
Small bowel polyp (including Peutz-Jegher disease)	10
Colonic tumor	1
Diverticula (n = 15)	
Ileum diverticulum	8
Meckel diverticulum	7
Other findings (n = 23)	
Cause not available	8
Anastomotic cause (ulcerated stenosis, cholecystojejunal, pancreas anastomotic disruption)	4
Chronic small bowel ischemia	2
Radiotherapy-induced small bowel lesions	2
Aberrant pancreas (whitish raised lesion in jejunum)	1
Amyloid lesion	1
Aortoenteral fistula	1
Henoch-Schönlein purpura	1
Hypertensive enteropathy	1
Ileal nevuslike lesion	1
Polyarteritis nodosa	1
Nondiagnostic (n = 97)	

Table 2
Operative management and results of intraoperative enteroscopy

	No. of Patients	Type of IOE (n)	Diagnostic Yield (%)	Therapeutic Yield (%)	Type of Treatment				Overall Morbidity (%)	Mortality (%)	Recurrent GI Bleeding (%)
					Surgical	Endoscopic	Combined	None			
Flickinger et al,[18] 1989	14	Transanally + enterotomy (14)	93	93	14	0	0	0	29	0	29
Lau,[21] 1990	17	Orally + transanally (17)	100	NA	NA	NA	NA	NA	24	18	0
Lewis et al,[10] 1991	23	Orally (23)	74	48	21	1	0	1	NA	4	39
Desa et al,[9] 1991	12	Orally (10), transanally (1), enterotomy (1)	83	83	12	0	0	0	50	17	25
Szold et al,[17] 1992	30	Orally (30)	93	93	30	0	0	0	NA	NA	NA
Ress et al,[23] 1992	44	Orally (31), transanally (4), via ileostomy (1), enterotomy (8)	70	70	31	1	2	10	16	11	52
Lopez et al,[22] 1996	16	Orally (16)	94	94	14	0	0	2	13	0	13
Lala et al,[20] 1998	12	Enterotomy (12)	75	75	NA	NA	NA	NA	NA	0	NA
Zaman et al,[16] 1999	12	Orally (12)	58	58	7	0	0	0	33	0	50
Douard et al,[2] 2000	25	Enterotomy (18), orally (5), orally + enterotomy (2)	60	84	20	0	0	5	16	4	24
Kendrick et al,[11] 2001	70	Enterotomy (70)	74	50	56	0	0	0	26	6	31

(continued on next page)

Table 2
(continued)

No. of Patients	Type of IOE (n)	Diagnostic Yield (%)	Therapeutic Yield (%)	Type of Treatment				Overall Morbidity (%)	Mortality (%)	Recurrent GI Bleeding (%)
				Surgical	Endoscopic	Combined	None			
Hartmann et al,[14,26] 2005, 2007	47	Enterotomy (47)	72	72	17	17	0	13	NA	2	26[a]
Jakobs et al,[19] 2006	81	Enterotomy (81)	84	84	24	20	24	13	1	0	NA
Kopáčová et al,[15] 2007	28	Enterotomy (28)	96	89	14	9	2	3	NA	7	14
Douard et al,[3] 2009	18[b]	Orally (6), orally + enterotomy (10), transanally (1), combined approaches (3)	67	67	13	4	0	1	33	11	17
Monsanto et al,[1] 2012	19[c]	Orally (6), orally + transanally (2), enterotomy (13)	79	78	12	1	1	4	21	5	21
Totals and mean values (range)	468		79.0 (58–100)	74.1 (48–94)					18 (1–50)	5 (0–18)	

Abbreviation: NA, not appreciated.

[a] Long-term follow-up reported a 26% rebleeding rate (Hartman et al,[26] 2007).
[b] Repeat IOE was performed in 2 patients.
[c] IOE was performed 3 times in one patient.

In addition to identifying hemorrhagic lesions, IOE allowed treatment in 74.1% of patients. The treatment was mainly surgery in the older studies and then was gradually superseded by endoscopic management alone or combined with surgery, as reported in **Table 2**.

These results were observed with the vascular lesions for which the proportions of surgical and endoscopic treatments were reversed between the first[2,3,9,10,16–18,22,23] and last studies.[3,14,19] Indeed, surgical resection of vascular lesions decreased from 96% of cases for the first studies to 12.5% of cases for the more recent studies, whereas endoscopic treatment alone increased from 2% of cases to 54.2% of cases, and combined endoscopic and surgical treatments increased from 2% of cases to 33.3% of cases. The ability of IOE to identify bleeding lesions is good and has been shown to be equal to the VCE diagnostic yield with a higher sensitivity than push-pull enteroscopy.[14]

However, diagnostic yield of the IOE, comparable to noninvasive explorations, does not mean that IOE has to be used as a diagnostic tool. When the bleeding site has not been formally preoperatively localized in the small bowel, IOE might be negative and/or bleeding sites may be discovered[1,3] outside the small bowel. For these reasons, some investigators decided to avoid IOE when a bleeding site has not been shown preoperatively in the small bowel. IOE has to be used to complete preoperative exploration, not to replace it.

Recurrent Gastrointestinal Bleeding

Recurrence of bleeding after IOE for obscure GI bleeding is reported in 13% to 52% of the cases (see **Table 2**). The yearly bleeding recurrence rate, which is calculated from $p = 1 - e(-rt)$, in which r is the rate and t is the time,[27] ranged from 12% to 60%.[1,3,9,11,16,22,23] This high rate is due to the predominance of vascular lesions in the causes of obscure GI bleeding and high rate of recurrence associated with these lesions.

These lesions are difficult to identify endoscopically because of possible confusion with lesions induced by endoscopy itself, as reported by Douard and colleagues.[2,3] In addition, part of rebleeding may be explained by the evanescence of these vascular lesions as mentioned by Gerson,[27] leading some investigators to propose an early deep enteroscopy exploration after OGIB.[28] Hartmann and colleagues[26] reported a recurrence rate of 26% after IOE with a single long-term follow-up. This high recurrence rate could be related to (i) the development of new lesions, (ii) the bleeding of missed lesions in the small bowel or other parts of the GI tract, and (iii) the real recurrence of the treated lesions.

This high rebleeding rate is in favor of endoscopic treatment of lesions identified during IOE in order to avoid the morbidity of surgical resection of small bowel with acceptable efficiency. Thus, the endoscopic treatment of angiodysplasia has been shown to reduce blood loss over long-term follow-up.[29,30] However, these results are disputed by some investigators who did not find any difference between endoscopic treatment and no treatment.[31,32] These therapeutic difficulties are especially present in elderly individuals with cardiovascular risks who are treated with antiaggregating medications and have higher risks for vascular lesions and bleeding. Nevertheless, the choice between surgical or endoscopic treatments remains debatable. In the authors' experience, the high recurrence rate of angiodysplasia that is endoscopically treated during IOE suggests that surgical resection of angiodysplasia could be proposed when a bleeding site has been clearly identified for localized lesions that are only reachable under IOE guidance.[3] In such cases, a recurrence at the same bleeding site would necessitate a second IOE to guide re-treatment.

What Is the Morbidity and Mortality of Intraoperative Enteroscopy?

IOE is associated with high morbidity and mortality, which has to be taken into account before proposing such technique. Morbidities of 1% to 50% have been reported in the literature (see **Table 2**). In studies with available data (11 studies that included 328 patients), overall morbidity affects 18% (n = 60) of the patients, including surgical morbidity, 12.5% (n = 41), and medical morbidity, 4.6% (n = 15).

The main causes of surgical morbidity are listed in **Table 3** and classified into 3 categories: mechanical causes, infectious causes, and hemorrhagic causes. Among these complications, the most common complication is postoperative ileus that was found in 20 patients (49% of all complications). The observed medical complications were pneumonia (n = 5), heart complications (n = 8), pulmonary embolism (n = 1), and azotemia (n = 1).

Mortality related to the procedure or to postoperative complications has been as high as 18% in some of the studies (see **Table 2**). Analysis of the 15 studies with available data (including 438 patients) showed an overall mortality associated with IOE of 5% (n = 22), which appears to be primarily related to multisystem organ failure with GI bleeding recurrence and septic causes (**Table 4**). Among the 15 series of significant size and using IOE, there were no laparoscopic series even if laparoscopic series of IOE have been published for other indications.[8]

Table 3
Overall morbidity (surgical and medical) in the 16 series

Overall Morbidity	No. of Patients
Surgical morbidity	
Mechanical causes	
Prolonged postoperative ileus	20
Small bowel obstruction	5
Bowel obstruction on pod 2 (repeat laparotomy)	1
Ventral hernia	1
Infectious causes	
Wound infection	4
Intra-abdominal abscess (1 suture leakage leading to reoperation, 1 operative drainage, 1 ultrasound drainage)	3
Colonic fistula	1
Douglas abscess (transrectal drainage)	1
Parietal infection	1
Hemorrhagic cause	
Hemorrhage from mesenteric bleeding (relaparotomy)	1
Hematochezia (suture line bleed: no specific treatment)	1
Hematemesis (caused by stress ulceration)	1
Nasogastric tube trauma (requiring transfusion)	1
Medical morbidity	
Pulmonary complication infection	5
Cardiac complications	8
Pulmonary embolism	1
Azotemia	1

Table 4
Mortality of the 16 series

Mortality	No. of Patients
Multisystem organ failure (with GI bleeding recurrence, n = 6)	7
Chest infection	2
Advanced neoplasia (extensive intestinal lymphoma)	2
Septic shock	2
Peritonitis (small bowel fistula)	1
Diffuse intravascular coagulopathy (with GI bleeding recurrence)	1
Cardiac arrhythmia (with GI bleeding recurrence)	1
Acute leukemic crisis (with GI bleeding recurrence)	1
Posthemorrhagic shock	1
Repeated episode of serious GI bleeding	2
Chronic renal failure (late death)	1
Cytomegalovirus enteritis	1
Small bowel ischemia	1
Unrelated cause	1

What Is the Remaining Role of Intraoperative Enteroscopy in the Exploration of Obscure Gastrointestinal Bleeding?

IOE has long been the only technical exploration of the entire small intestine available, especially in cases of digestive occult bleeding. However, due to its high morbidity and mortality, IOE has been gradually replaced by less invasive exploration techniques and/or procedures associated with less morbidity. Among these new techniques, VCE is the least invasive method to explore the entire small bowel and to diagnose hemorrhagic lesions with good accuracy. Thus, in a prospective study that compares VCE and IOE, the sensitivity and specificity of VCE were 95% and 75%, respectively, with positive and negative predictive values of 95% and 86%, respectively.[14] Because of these results, many guidelines recommend performing a VCE as an initial diagnostic test in cases of OGIB after negative upper endoscopy and colonoscopy.[3,14,33] However, 20% tumor miss rates and incomplete small bowel visualization rates have been reported with VCE,[34] in addition to other limitations, such as no maneuverability, no therapeutic capabilities, and the risk of retention by strictures.

New techniques of enteroscopy were also developed in order to explore more consistently and specifically all of the parts of the small bowel with the opportunity to combine therapeutic procedure with diagnostic procedure. These techniques include balloon-assisted endoscopy using either 2 balloons (double-balloon enteroscopy), 1 balloon (single-balloon enteroscopy), or balloon-guided enteroscopy and spiral enteroscopy. Compared with single enteroscopy (named also push enteroscopy), the double-balloon enteroscopy technique increases the length of procedure and diagnostic yield.[35,36] Double-balloon enteroscopy allows visualization of the entire small bowel in 40% to 80% of cases[36–39] and appears to be superior to the simple enteroscopy that allows a complete visualization of the small bowel in only 5% to 25% of cases.[40,41] Spiral enteroscopy has recently been described[41] and could reduce the examination time.[42] However, more experience is needed to confirm the safety and potential superiority of spiral enteroscopy to single-balloon enteroscopy. Comparative studies between deep enteroscopy techniques are scarce. Double-balloon enteroscopy appears to allow more bowel to be visualized compared with single-balloon enteroscopy[37] and at least as much as spiral enteroscopy.[43,44] Moreover, it has been shown that VCE and double-balloon enteroscopy provide similar diagnostic yield results in small bowel disease, including OGIB.[45]

Following all of these publications, it is clear that the VCE and balloon-assisted endoscopy have supplanted simple enteroscopy as first-line exploration method for occult GI bleeding. In addition, balloon-assisted enteroscopy (with 1 or 2 balloons) allows combination of therapeutic treatment with diagnostic exploration. The negative predictive value of these techniques is so high that some investigators recommend repeating conventional upper endoscopy and colonoscopy in the case of negativity of VCE or balloon-assisted endoscopy.[3] This recommendation is supported by cases of gastric Dieulafoy lesions that had been missed in the preoperative endoscopic workup before IOE.[2] When the small bowel lesion cannot be treated during deep enteroscopy, tattoo marks have been proposed to guide surgical treatment. Consequently, IOE is avoided as a first-line localization tool.[12]

In parallel with the development of endoscopic techniques, vascular and radiological studies have evolved to provide additional information in the preoperative staging of occult GI bleeding. Therefore, although endoscopic explorations reveal potential mucosal lesions, contrast studies have low sensitivity to these same lesions such as small angiodysplasia.[46,47] On the contrary, these techniques of vascular explorations have a high sensitivity to the parietal lesions, such as stenosis caused by inflammatory bowel diseases or neoplasms,[48] which can be surgically treated without any preoperative endoscopic exploration.

Small bowel follow-through has now been superseded by computed tomography enterography, and more recently, by magnetic resonance enterography (MRE) in these indications.[49–51] Vascular explorations, such as computed tomography angiography and angiography, are used to assess vascular lesions, such as angiodysplasia, that are frequently reported in obscure GI bleeding. Computed tomography angiography and angiography are good methods of locating the bleeding site during an active hemorrhage. In this indication, computed tomography angiography is the first-line examination and could guide a subsequent selective conventional angiography to perform selective embolization.[52] Provocative testing has been recently proposed to increase the diagnostic yield of endoscopic and/or angiographic explorations, but data are lacking on the risks and benefits.[53]

The diagnostic and therapeutic management for OGIB depends on both hemodynamic impact of this bleeding, but also the expertise of endoscopists, radiologists, surgeons, and interventional radiologists of the hospital where the patient is located. Because of the high negative predictive value of deep enteroscopy and/or VCE in the localizing bleeding lesions in the small bowel, the authors think that IOE has to be avoided as a diagnostic tool in the evaluation of obscure GI bleeding.

Nevertheless, apart from obscure GI bleeding exploration, IOE seems to keep a wide indication in inherited polyposis syndromes such as familial adenomatous polyposis (FAP) and Peutz-Jeghers syndrome (PJS).

In the FAP, the reference examination for the proximal small bowel is the conventional forward-viewing and side-viewing endoscopy due to the high cumulative risk of severe duodenal polyposis and high relative risk of duodenal cancer. Nevertheless, jejunal and ileal polyps can be also found in 40% to 70% of FAP patients, specifically in patients with severe duodenal polyposis.[54] In these cases, VCE has demonstrated higher sensitivity to diagnose jejunal and ileal polyp than radiological investigation,[55] and studies comparing push-enteroscopy with VCE have shown conflicting results.[56] However, when a polyp larger than 1 cm is identified by VCE or radiological investigation, an enteroscopy is indicated to obtain targeted biopsies and accomplish endoscopic polypectomy.

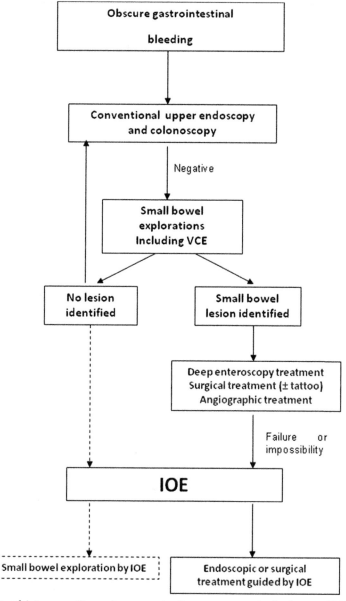

Fig. 2. Place of intraoperative enteroscopy in the management of obscure GI bleeding. (*Adapted from* Bonnet S, Douard R, Malamut G, et al. Intraoperative enteroscopy in the management of obscure gastrointestinal bleeding. Dig Liver Dis 2013;45:279; with permission.)

Similarly, in PJS patients, there is a high risk of polyp-burden and polyp-related complications, such as intussusception and occult hemorrhage requiring small-bowel surveillance and large polyp resection. In these cases, radiological examinations such as MRE are recommended as first line for small bowel surveillance in order to limit the risk of obstruction by VCE in large polyps. MRE was also shown to be less prone to missing large polyps than VCE.[57] When large polyps (>10–15 mm) are discovered by radiological examination, an enteroscopy with polypectomy is required.

In FAP and PJS, the choice for the type of enteroscopy is especially guided by patient's surgical history. An IOE will be preferred in patients with FAP in whom a Whipple procedure with a Roux-en-Y anastomosis has been performed. Similarly, in FAP or PJS, completeness of small bowel investigation by balloon-assisted enteroscopy may be compromised by previous laparotomies due to multiple adhesions, and IOE will then be preferred. IOE has been demonstrated to enhance small bowel clearance and to reduce the number of laparotomies.[58]

Overall, when noninvasive techniques are unavailable, are unable to explore the entire small bowel, or have conflicting results, IOE may still have a place.[1] However, IOE may be used to guide surgical or endoscopic treatment when small bowel lesions have been demonstrated preoperatively. In the authors' opinion, IOE remains indicated in some cases when small bowel lesions (i) have been identified by a preoperative workup (VCE, balloon-assisted endoscopy, and/or other explorations such as angiography), (ii) cannot be definitively managed by angiographic embolization or endoscopic treatment with deep enteroscopy or when surgery is required for other reasons, and (iii) cannot be localized during surgical explorations (ie, no serosal visible lesion and/or no previous tattoo) (**Fig. 2**). In such conditions, IOE allows intraoperative localization of preoperatively determined lesions and appropriate concomitant treatment. For certain indications, laparoscopic-assisted IOE might be proposed to reduce the morbidity of conventional procedures.[40–43,59]

SUMMARY

The diagnostic and therapeutic management for OGIB depends on both hemodynamic impact of this bleeding and the expertise of endoscopists, radiologists, surgeons, and interventional radiologists of the hospital where the patient is located. Because of the high negative predictive value of deep enteroscopy and/or VCE in the localizing bleeding lesions in the small bowel, the authors think that IOE has to be avoided as a diagnostic tool in the evaluation of obscure GI bleeding. Nevertheless, when noninvasive techniques are unavailable, are unable to explore the entire small bowel, or have conflicting results, IOE could still have a place.[1] However, IOE may be used to guide to surgical or endoscopic treatment when small bowel lesions have been demonstrated preoperatively. In the authors' opinion, IOE remains indicated in some cases when small bowel lesions (i) have been identified by a preoperative workup (VCE, balloon-assisted endoscopy, and/or other explorations such as angiography), (ii) cannot be definitively managed by angiographic embolization or endoscopic treatment with deep enteroscopy or when surgery is required for other reasons, and (iii) cannot be localized during surgical explorations (ie, no serosal visible lesion and/or no previous tattoo) (see **Fig. 2**). In such conditions, IOE allows intraoperative localization of preoperatively determined lesions and appropriate concomitant treatment. For certain indications, laparoscopic-assisted IOE might be proposed to reduce the morbidity of conventional procedures.[40–43,59]

In rare cases when preoperative techniques are not available or have conflicting results or when a GI bleeding site has not been preoperatively localized, IOE could still be used as a diagnostic tool. Such indications have to be used with caution, because of the risk of negative IOE with the intraoperative discover of bleeding sites outside of the small bowel. In such situations, the performance of IOE after treatment of another bleeding site must be counterbalanced with induced morbidity.

Apart from obscure GI bleeding exploration, IOE remains indicated in FAP and PJS to enhance polyp clearance and reduce the number of laparotomies,[58] especially in patients with a complex past surgical history (Whipple procedure, previous laparotomies) for whom a complete exploration of the small bowel by other techniques would be compromised.

REFERENCES

1. Monsanto P, Almeida N, Lérias C, et al. Is there still a role for intraoperative enteroscopy in patients with obscure gastrointestinal bleeding? Rev Esp Enferm Dig 2012;104:190–6.
2. Douard R, Wind P, Panis Y, et al. Intraoperative enteroscopy for diagnosis and management of unexplained gastrointestinal bleeding. Am J Surg 2000;180:181–4.
3. Douard R, Wind P, Berger A, et al. Role of intraoperative enteroscopy in the management of obscure gastointestinal bleeding at the time of video-capsule endoscopy. Am J Surg 2009;198:6–11.
4. Reddy ND, Rao VG. Laparoscopically assisted panenteroscopy for snare excision. Gastrointest Endosc 1996;44:208–9.
5. Agarwal A. Use of the laparoscope to perform intraoperative enteroscopy. Surg Endosc 1999;13:1143–4.
6. Ingrosso M, Prete F, Pisani A, et al. Laparoscopically assisted total enteroscopy: a new approach to small intestinal diseases. Gastrointest Endosc 1999;49:651–3.
7. Sriram PV, Rao GV, Reddy DN. Laparoscopically assisted panenteroscopy. Gastrointest Endosc 2001;54:805–6.
8. Hotokezaka M, Jimi S, Hidaka H, et al. Intraoperative enteroscopy in minimally invasive surgery. Surg Laparosc Endosc Percutan Tech 2007;17:492–4.
9. Desa LA, Ohri SK, Hutton KA, et al. Role of intraoperative enteroscopy in obscure gastrointestinal bleeding of small bowel origin. Br J Surg 1991;78:192–5.
10. Lewis BS, Wenger JS, Waye JD. Small bowel enteroscopy and intraoperative enteroscopy for obscure gastrointestinal bleeding. Am J Gastroenterol 1991;86:171–4.
11. Kendrick ML, Buttar NS, Anderson MA, et al. Contribution of intraoperative enteroscopy in the management of obscure gastrointestinal bleeding. J Gastrointest Surg 2001;5:162–7.
12. Konishi H, Kikuchi S, Miyashita A, et al. Minimally invasive surgery for obscure idiopathic ileal varices diagnosed by capsule endoscopy and double balloon endoscopy: report of a case. Surg Today 2010;40:1088–92.
13. Pontone S, Pironi D, Arcieri S, et al. Intraoperative enteroscopy by standard colonoscope with a minimal contamination technique. Surg Laparosc Endosc Percutan Tech 2013;23:e11–3.
14. Hartmann D, Schmidt H, Bolz G, et al. A prospective two-center study comparing wireless capsule endoscopy with intraoperative enteroscopy in patients with obscure GI bleeding. Gastrointest Endosc 2005;61:826–32.
15. Kopácová M, Bures J, Vykouril L, et al. Intraoperative enteroscopy: ten years' experience at a single tertiary center. Surg Endosc 2007;21:1111–6.
16. Zaman A, Sheppard B, Katon RM. Total peroral intraoperative enteroscopy for obscure GI bleeding using a dedicated push enteroscope: diagnostic yield and patient outcome. Gastrointest Endosc 1999;50:506–10.
17. Szold A, Katz LB, Lewis BS. Surgical approach to occult gastrointestinal bleeding. Am J Surg 1992;163:90–3.
18. Flickinger EG, Stanforth AC, Sinar DR, et al. Intraoperative video panendoscopy for diagnosing sites of chronic intestinal bleeding. Am J Surg 1989;157:137–44.

19. Jakobs R, Hartmann D, Benz C, et al. Diagnosis of obscure gastrointestinal bleeding by intra-operative enteroscopy in 81 consecutive patients. World J Gastroenterol 2006;12:313–6.

20. Lala AK, Sitaram V, Perakath B, et al. Intraoperative enteroscopy in obscure gastrointestinal hemorrhage. Hepatogastroenterology 1998;45:597–602.

21. Lau WY. Intraoperative enteroscopy–indications and limitations. Gastrointest Endosc 1990;36:268–71.

22. Lopez MJ, Cooley JS, Petros JG, et al. Complete intraoperative small-bowel endoscopy in the evaluation of occult gastrointestinal bleeding using the sonde enteroscope. Arch Surg 1996;131:272–7.

23. Ress AM, Benacci JC, Sarr MG. Efficacy of intraoperative enteroscopy in diagnosis and prevention of recurrent, occult gastrointestinal bleeding. Am J Surg 1992;163:94–8.

24. Pennazio M. Enteroscopy in the diagnosis and management of obscure gastrointestinal bleeding. Gastrointest Endosc Clin N Am 2009;19:409–26.

25. Van Gossum A. Obscure digestive bleeding. Best Pract Res Clin Gastroenterol 2001;15:155–74.

26. Hartmann D, Schmidt H, Schilling D, et al. Follow-up of patients with obscure gastrointestinal bleeding after capsule endoscopy and intraoperative enteroscopy. Hepatogastroenterology 2007;54:780–3.

27. Gerson LB. Outcomes associated with deep enteroscopy. Gastrointest Endosc Clin N Am 2009;19:481–96.

28. Shinozaki S, Yamamoto H, Yano T, et al. Long-term outcome of patients with obscure gastrointestinal bleeding investigated by double-balloon endoscopy. Clin Gastroenterol Hepatol 2010;8:151–8.

29. Vakil N, Huilgol V, Khan I. Effect of push enteroscopy on transfusion requirements and quality of life in patients with unexplained gastrointestinal bleeding. Am J Gastroenterol 1997;92:425–8.

30. Morris AJ, Mokhashi M, Straiton M, et al. Push enteroscopy and heater probe therapy for small bowel bleeding. Gastrointest Endosc 1996;44:394–7.

31. Schmit A, Gay F, Adler M, et al. Diagnostic efficacy of push-enteroscopy and long-term follow-up of patients with small bowel angiodysplasias. Dig Dis Sci 1996;41:2348–52.

32. Lewis BS, Kornbluth A. Hormonal therapy for bleeding from angiodysplasia: chronic renal failure, et al? Am J Gastroenterol 1990;85:1649–51.

33. Raju GS, Gerson L, Das A, et al. American Gastroenterological Association (AGA) Institute technical review on obscure gastrointestinal bleeding. Gastroenterology 2007;133:1697–717.

34. Lewis BS, Eisen GM, Friedman S. A pooled analysis to evaluate results of capsule endoscopy trials. Endoscopy 2005;37:960–5.

35. Mehdizadeh S, Han NJ, Cheng DW, et al. Success rate of retrograde double-balloon enteroscopy. Gastrointest Endosc 2007;65:633–9.

36. May A, Färber M, Aschmoneit I, et al. Prospective multicenter trial comparing push-and-pull enteroscopy with the single- and double-balloon techniques in patients with small-bowel disorders. Am J Gastroenterol 2010;105:575–81.

37. Takano N, Yamada A, Watabe H, et al. Single-balloon versus double-balloon endoscopy for achieving total enteroscopy: a randomized, controlled trial. Gastrointest Endosc 2011;73:734–9.

38. Pohl J, Blancas JM, Cave D, et al. Consensus report of the 2nd International Conference on double balloon endoscopy. Endoscopy 2008;40:156–60.

39. May A. How much importance do we have to place on complete enteroscopy? Gastrointest Endosc 2011;73:740–3.

40. Ramchandani M, Reddy DN, Gupta R, et al. Diagnostic yield and therapeutic impact of single-balloon enteroscopy: series of 106 cases. J Gastroenterol Hepatol 2009;24:1631–8.

41. Buscaglia JM, Okolo PI 3rd. Deep enteroscopy: training, indications, and the endoscopic technique. Gastrointest Endosc 2011;73:1023–8.

42. May A, Manner H, Aschmoneit I, et al. Prospective, cross-over, single-center trial comparing oral double-balloon enteroscopy and oral spiral enteroscopy in patients with suspected small-bowel vascular malformations. Endoscopy 2011;43: 477–83.

43. Khashab MA, Lennon AM, Dunbar KB, et al. A comparative evaluation of single-balloon enteroscopy and spiral enteroscopy for patients with mid-gut disorders. Gastrointest Endosc 2010;72:766–72.

44. Frieling T, Heise J, Sassenrath W, et al. Prospective comparison between double-balloon enteroscopy and spiral enteroscopy. Endoscopy 2010;42:885–8.

45. Pasha SF, Leighton JA, Das A, et al. Double-balloon enteroscopy and capsule endoscopy have comparable diagnostic yield in small-bowel disease: a meta-analysis. Clin Gastroenterol Hepatol 2008;6:671–6.

46. Fried AM, Poulos A, Hatfield DR. The effectiveness of the incidental small-bowel series. Radiology 1981;140:45–6.

47. Rabe FE, Becker GJ, Besozzi MJ, et al. Efficacy study of the small-bowel examination. Radiology 1981;140:47–50.

48. Korman U, Kantarci F, Selçuk D, et al. Enteroclysis in obscure gastrointestinal system hemorrhage of small bowel origin. Turk J Gastroenterol 2003;14:243–9.

49. Fiorino G, Bonifacio C, Peyrin-Biroulet L, et al. Prospective comparison of computed tomography enterography and magnetic resonance enterography for assessment of disease activity and complications in ileocolonic Crohn's disease. Inflamm Bowel Dis 2011;17:1073–80.

50. Jensen MD, Kjeldsen J, Rafaelsen SR, et al. Diagnostic accuracies of MR enterography and CT enterography in symptomatic Crohn's disease. Scand J Gastroenterol 2011;46:1449–57.

51. He B, Gong S, Hu C, et al. Obscure gastrointestinal bleeding: diagnostic performance of 64-section multiphase CT enterography and CT angiography compared with capsule endoscopy. Br J Radiol 2014;87:20140229.

52. Ettorre GC, Francioso G, Garribba AP, et al. Helical CT angiography in gastrointestinal bleeding of obscure origin. AJR Am J Roentgenol 1997;168:727–31.

53. Mernagh JR, O'Donovan N, Somers S, et al. Use of heparin in the investigation of obscure gastrointestinal bleeding. Can Assoc Radiol J 2001;52:232–5.

54. Jagelman DG, DeCosse JJ, Bussey HJ. Upper gastrointestinal cancer in familial adenomatous polyposis. Lancet 1988;1:1149–51.

55. Schulmann K, Hollerbach S, Kraus K, et al. Feasibility and diagnostic utility of video capsule endoscopy for the detection of small bowel polyps in patients with hereditary polyposis syndromes. Am J Gastroenterol 2005;100:27–37.

56. Wong RF, Tuteja AK, Haslem DS, et al. Video capsule endoscopy compared with standard endoscopy for the evaluation of small-bowel polyps in persons with familial adenomatous polyposis (with video). Gastrointest Endosc 2006;64:530–7.

57. Gupta A, Postgate AJ, Burling D, et al. A prospective study of MR enterography versus capsule endoscopy for the surveillance of adult patients with Peutz-Jeghers syndrome. AJR Am J Roentgenol 2010;195:108–16.

58. Edwards DP, Khosraviani K, Stafferton R, et al. Long-term results of polyp clearance by intraoperative enteroscopy in the Peutz-Jeghers syndrome. Dis Colon Rectum 2003;46:48–50.
59. Aktas H, de Ridder L, Haringsma J, et al. Complications of single-balloon enteroscopy: a prospective evaluation of 166 procedures. Endoscopy 2010;42:365–8.

Small Bowel Bleeding
Updated Algorithm and Outcomes

Lauren B. Gerson, MD, MSc

KEYWORDS

- Suspected small bowel hemorrhage • Obscure GI bleeding
- Video capsule endoscopy • Deep enteroscopy • Angiography

KEY POINTS

- Video capsule endoscopy (VCE) should be the third diagnostic test after routine upper and lower endoscopic examinations.
- Computed tomographic enterography or magnetic resonance enterography (MRE) examinations should be performed in patients with suspected small bowel strictures from nonsteroidal anti-inflammatory agents, inflammatory bowel disease, prior radiation, or after normal VCE examinations.
- Patients with abnormal findings on small bowel imaging should be treated using deep enteroscopy, angiography, or surgery.
- For patients with ongoing bleeding or anemia and negative testing should undergo repeated testing with VCE, enteroscopy, or other testing until a source is identified.
- The algorithms for patients with overt and/or occult suspected small bowel bleeding are equivalent.

INTRODUCTION

Formerly classified as "obscure [gastrointestinal] GI bleeding," this diagnostic term has been replaced by "suspected small bowel bleeding" or "small bowel bleeding" in the recent 2015 American College of Gastroenterology (ACG) guidelines.[1] The reason for this change in classification is because most bleeding sources outside the upper or lower digestive tracts are found within the small intestine on further investigation with video capsule endoscopy (VCE), deep enteroscopy, computed tomography enterography (CTE), or magnetic resonance enterography (MRE) examinations. This article provides clinicians with algorithms for how to manage patients with suspected small bowel bleeding.

Disclosure Statement: Dr L.B. Gerson is a consultant for Capsovision, Inc and Olympus America, Inc.

Division of Gastroenterology, Department of Medicine, California Pacific Medical Center, University of California, San Francisco, 2340 Clay Street, 6th Floor, San Francisco, CA 94115, USA
E-mail address: lgersonmd@yahoo.com

An initial algorithm for patients with obscure GI bleeding developed at the International Conference on Capsule Endoscopy (ICCE) conference in 2005 was published by Pennazio and colleagues[2] and is shown in **Fig. 1**. An important recommendation of all algorithms to date has been the consideration for second-look endoscopic examinations before proceeding with VCE. The rationale for this recommendation has that second-look examinations, particularly upper endoscopic examinations, have been associated with diagnostic yields ranging from 3% to 60%, as shown in **Table 1**. These numbers were derived from patients undergoing push enteroscopy, VCE, or deep enteroscopy. The most common lesions found on repeat examinations were angiodysplastic lesions. The algorithms presented in this article were recently published in the updated 2015 ACG guideline "Management of Small Bowel Bleeding."

Summary Algorithm

As shown in **Fig. 1**, patients may present with overt (melena or hematochezia) or occult (iron-deficiency anemia with or without heme-positive stools) suspected small bowel bleeding. The first step that the clinician needs to take is whether to repeat upper and or lower endoscopic examinations. This decision is based on a variety of factors, including the date of the prior examination and the quality of the prior examination, whether there was blood present in the upper tract, and the quality of the bowel preparation. If the patient did not have an examination of the upper tract within the preceding 2 to 3 months and presents with symptoms suggesting of upper GI bleeding, it is not unreasonable to repeat an upper endoscopy. Data regarding the diagnostic yield

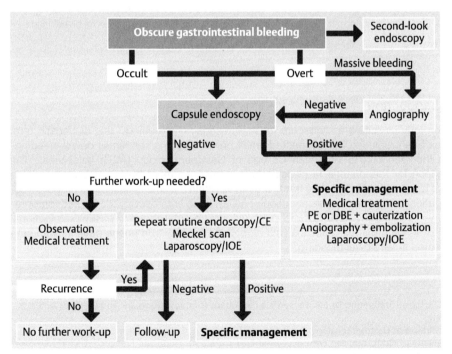

Fig. 1. 2005 Management algorithm for obscure GI bleeding. CE, capsule endoscopy; DBE, double-balloon enteroscopy; IOE, intraoperative enteroscopy; PE, push enteroscopy. (*Data from* Pennazio M, Eisen G, Goldfarb N; ICCE. ICCE consensus for obscure gastrointestinal bleeding. Endoscopy 2005;37:1046–50; with permission.)

Table 1
Yield of second-look examinations before video capsule endoscopy cam

Author, Year	Modality	Number of Subjects, Diagnostic Yield (%)	EGD or Colonoscopy (Colon), Yield (%)	Most Common Findings
Zaman & Katon,[13] 1998	PE	95 (41%)	EGD: 25 (64%)	Upper source: Cameron ulcerations (N = 8) Gastric AVMs (N = 5) Duodenum: AVMs (N = 7) Jejunum: AVMs (N = 6)
Descamps et al,[14] 1999	PE	233 (53%)	EGD: 25 (10%)	Cameron ulcerations (N = 6) GU (N = 5) DU (N = 1) GJ anastomosis (N = 1) Gastric angiodysplasia (N = 5) Duodenal angiodysplasia (N = 4) Duodenal tumor (N = 1) Hemosuccus pancreaticus (N = 2)
Lara et al,[15] 2005	PE	35 (56%)	EGD: 10 (59%)	GU (N = 2) Esophageal varices (N = 2) DU (N = 1) Gastric remnant (N = 1) Gastric AVM (N = 2) Cameron ulcerations (N = 2)

(continued on next page)

Table 1
(continued)

Author, Year	Modality	Number of Subjects, Diagnostic Yield (%)	EGD or Colonoscopy (Colon), Yield (%)	Most Common Findings
Fry et al,[16] 2009	DBE	107 (65%)	EGD: 13 (12%) Colon: 12 (11%)	Upper source: GU (n = 3) DU (n = 4) Cameron lesions (n = 2) GAVE (n = 4) Duodenal AVM (n = 1) GAVE (N = 1) Erosive esophagitis (N = 1) Lower source: Radiation proctitis (n = 1) Radiation ileitis (n = 2) Hemorrhoids with stigmata of recent bleed (n = 1) Colon angiodysplasias (n = 3) Colon diverticulosis (n = 3) Colonic Crohn disease (n = 1) Anastomotic ulcers (n = 1)
Van Turenhout et al,[17] 2010	VCE	592 (49%)	EGD: 32 (17%) Colon: 8 (4%)	Upper source: Gastritis or erosions (N = 24) GU (N = 5) Hematin (N = 6) Blood (N = 5) Lower source: Colonic angioectasia (N = 6) Colonic erosions (N = 3) Blood in colon (N = 1)

| Lorenceau-Savale et al,[18] 2010 | VCE | 65 (57%) | EGD or colon: 8/35 (23%) | Upper source:
Gastric Dieulafoy N = 1)
Cameron ulcerations (N = 2)
Portal hypertensive gastropathy (N = 1)
Angioectasia (N = 2)
Lower source:
Colonic bleeding diverticulum (N = 1)
Angioectasia (N = 1) |
| Robinson et al,[19] 2011 | VCE | 707 (40%) | EGD: 22 (3%)
Colon: 6 (1%) | Upper source:
Erosive esophagitis (N = 7)
Portal hypertensive gastropathy (N = 5)
GU or DU (N = 4)
HH (N = 1)
Hiatal hernia (n = 1)
Blood in stomach (N = 1)
BE (N = 1)
GAVE (N = 3)
Lower source:
Diverticular bleeding (N = 1)
Colorectal cancer (N = 1)
Colonic AVM (N = 2)
Blood in the colon (N = 2) |

Abbreviations: AVM, arteriovenous malformation; BE, barrett's esophagus; DU, duodenal ulcer; EGD, upper endoscopy; GAVE, gastric antral vascular ectasia; GJ, gastrojejunal anastomosis; GU, gastric ulcer; HH, hiatal hernia.

associated with repeat upper examinations show diagnostic yields ranging from 25% to 60% (see **Table 1**). The most commonly missed lesions are angiodysplastic lesions and ulcerations.

In the 2005 algorithm that was proposed as part of the ICCE consensus conference and cited in the 2007 guidelines by the American Gastroenterological Association,[3] angiography is recommended in cases of massive overt bleeding. If the angiography is negative or if patients present with stable overt or occult bleeding, VCE is recommended as the third diagnostic test. The reason for this recommendation (see later discussion) is the ability of VCE to visualize the entire small bowel in more than 80% of cases, particularly now with 12-hour battery life and the noninvasive nature of the test. In a subsequent 2008 meta-analysis, VCE was shown to have a higher diagnostic rate compared with double-balloon enteroscopy.[4] In addition, performance of a deep enteroscopy after initial VCE has been shown to increase the diagnostic yield of the enteroscopy examination.[5]

In the 2005 algorithm and subsequent algorithms published in the 2015 ACG guidelines, the recommendation was to perform a therapeutic procedure if the VCE demonstrated an abnormal finding. Endoscopic therapy of small bowel angioectasia has been shown to reduce subsequent risk[4] of rebleeding. On the other hand, rebleeding rates from angioectasia have been shown to be significant, approaching 30% to 40% per year, particularly for patients who are at risk, including patients with Heyde syndrome[6] or renal failure.[7] In some of these patients with refractory bleeding or for elderly patients who are not candidates for endoscopic intervention, medical therapy with octreotide or thalidomide can be considered.[8]

On the other hand, for the patients with angioectasias who are no longer anemic, observation or treatment with iron has been recommended because 30% to 40% of patients with isolated lesions have been shown to have spontaneous cessation of bleeding without endoscopic therapy.[9]

In the 2015 ACG Guideline, the term obscure GI bleeding was replaced by the term small bowel bleeding, with the term obscure reserved for patients without a source identified on VCE, deep enteroscopy, or enterography examination. The reason for this change in terminology was related to several advancements: (1) the literature on repeat endoscopic examinations of the upper and/or lower tracts demonstrated findings in 30% to 40% of patients, (2) utilization of VCE or deep enteroscopy detected lesions in the small bowel in 50% to 60% of patients, and (3) in patients with normal VCE or enteroscopy examinations, disease is found on CTE or MRE in 40% to 50% of patients.

The algorithm for suspected small bowel bleeding from the 2015 guideline is shown in **Fig. 2**. Realizing that VCE retention can occur in approximately 1% to 2% of patients with small bowel bleeding and up to 5% to 10% of patients with suspected or established inflammatory bowel disease (IBD),[1] the new guidelines recommend imaging with CTE or MRE before VCE in patients with possible signs of obstruction. Radiographic imaging should occur in patients with abdominal pain, history of abdominal radiation, heavy use of nonsteroidal antiinflammatory drugs, or history of IBD. Use of the patency capsule, a capsule with a lactose body that dissolves into a radiofrequency identification tag, is another option instead of CTE or MRE for patients with suspected stricture. If the CTE or MRE is negative, then VCE is recommended with specific therapy if findings are identified. Use of intraoperative enteroscopy has been mainly replaced by deep enteroscopy, with the exception of patients with adhesions from prior surgeries that require surgical lysis to facilitate small bowel advancement. In patients with normal VCE examinations, recommendations are to proceed with CTE or MRE to evaluate for submucosal disease instead of deep enteroscopy, unless there is high clinical suspicion for small bowel angioectasia.

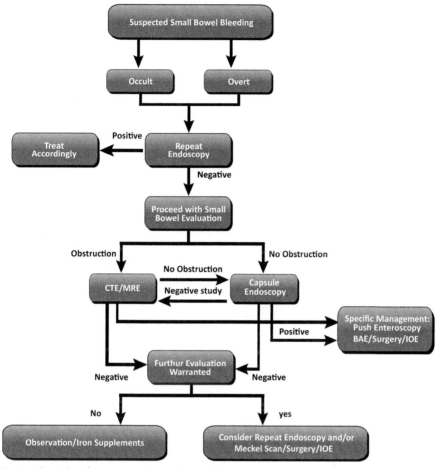

Fig. 2. Algorithm for suspected small bowel bleeding. BAE, balloon-assisted enteroscopy.

Patients at the end of the algorithm, who have undergone normal VCE, enteroscopy, and CTE or MRE examinations, can be considered to have obscure GI bleeding. Ongoing evaluation is recommended if patients have ongoing bleeding but the order of repeated testing has not been determined. In younger patients, Meckel's scans can be considered. The yield of repeat VCE is highest in the setting of repeated overt bleeding, drop in hemoglobin, and within 2 weeks of an overt bleeding episode.[10] The yield of repeat VCE has been shown to be as high as 50% to 75%. Similarly, the yield of VCE or deep enteroscopy has been shown to be highest within 2 weeks of an overt bleeding episode.[11]

For patients with massive suspected small bowel bleeding presenting with hemodynamic instability, the gastroenterologist should call interventional radiology (**Fig. 3**). A new addition since the 2005 guideline, computed tomography (CT) angiography is the preferred diagnostic modality of choice when available because it can help direct subsequent angiography and therapeutic embolization. A patient bleeding at a slower rate, 1 to 2 mL/minute, will be typically referred for tagged nuclear medicine red blood cell scans rather than angiography, in an attempt to localize the site of bleeding. For

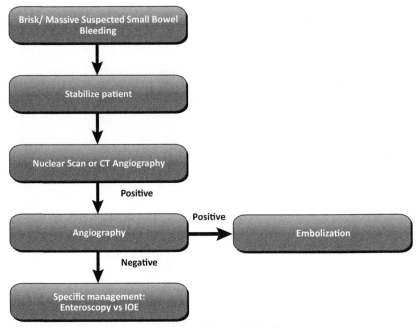

Fig. 3. Algorithm for massive suspected small bowel bleeding.

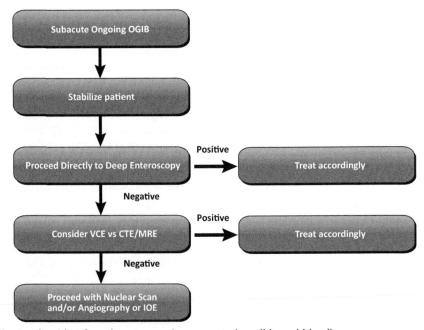

Fig. 4. Algorithm for subacute ongoing suspected small bowel bleeding.

patients with negative angiography, deep enteroscopy can be subsequently attempted for treatment.

As shown in **Fig. 4**, patients with stable ongoing overt bleeding can be considered to undergo direct deep enteroscopy because performance of VCE requires additional time to prepare patients with bowel preparation and to read the examination. If patients undergoing deep enteroscopy are from Western countries, the probability of finding lesions is higher in the proximal small bowel and an anterograde approach should be used.

For patients with occult suspected small bowel hemorrhage, the evaluation is equivalent to patients with overt hemorrhage but the diagnostic yield has been shown to be somewhat lower compared with patients with acute overt bleeding.[12]

SUMMARY

The diagnosis of small bowel bleeding has significantly advanced with the advent of VCE, deep enterography, and CTE or MRE examinations. Patients with IBD or risk of small bowel stricture should undergo enterography examination initially. In patients with massive bleeding, CT angiography should be the initial test in that in can guide subsequent angiography and embolization. In most patients, VCE should be the initial test with a bowel preparation because it can determine whether a small bowel lesion is present and the location of the lesion. When a pathologic finding is identified, deep enteroscopy should follow for therapy and/or further diagnosis. Intraoperative enteroscopy should be reserved for patients with adhesions requiring lysis or for patients with significant polyposis syndromes requiring extensive polypectomy. In most patients with small bowel bleeding in Western countries, a source will be identified using an anterograde approach; however, total enteroscopy should be performed when there is a high suspicion of a small bowel lesion.

REFERENCES

1. Gerson LB, Fidler JL, Cave DR, et al. ACG clinical guideline: diagnosis and management of small bowel bleeding. Am J Gastroenterol 2015;110:1265–87 [quiz: 1288].

2. Pennazio M, Eisen G, Goldfarb N. ICCE consensus for obscure gastrointestinal bleeding. Endoscopy 2005;37:1046–50.

3. Raju GS, Gerson L, Das A, et al. American Gastroenterological Association (AGA) institute technical review on obscure gastrointestinal bleeding. Gastroenterology 2007;133:1697–717.

4. Pasha SF, Leighton JA, Das A, et al. Double-balloon enteroscopy and capsule endoscopy have comparable diagnostic yield in small-bowel disease: a meta-analysis. Clin Gastroenterol Hepatol 2008;6:671–6.

5. Teshima CW, Kuipers EJ, van Zanten SV, et al. Double balloon enteroscopy and capsule endoscopy for obscure gastrointestinal bleeding: an updated meta-analysis. J Gastroenterol Hepatol 2011;26:796–801.

6. Batur P, Stewart WJ, Isaacson JH. Increased prevalence of aortic stenosis in patients with arteriovenous malformations of the gastrointestinal tract in Heyde syndrome. Arch Intern Med 2003;163:1821–4.

7. Lepere C, Cuillerier E, Van Gossum A, et al. Predictive factors of positive findings in patients explored by push enteroscopy for unexplained GI bleeding. Gastrointest Endosc 2005;61:709–14.

8. Jackson CS, Gerson LB. Management of gastrointestinal angiodysplastic lesions (GIADs): a systematic review and meta-analysis. Am J Gastroenterol 2014;109: 474–83.

9. Junquera F, Feu F, Papo M, et al. A multicenter, randomized, clinical trial of hormonal therapy in the prevention of rebleeding from gastrointestinal angiodysplasia. Gastroenterology 2001;121:1073–9.

10. Viazis N, Papaxoinis K, Vlachogiannakos J, et al. Is there a role for second-look capsule endoscopy in patients with obscure GI bleeding after a nondiagnostic first test? Gastrointest Endosc 2009;69:850–6.

11. Bresci G, Parisi G, Bertoni M, et al. The role of video capsule endoscopy for evaluating obscure gastrointestinal bleeding: usefulness of early use. J Gastroenterol 2005;40:256–9.

12. Pennazio M, Santucci R, Rondonotti E, et al. Outcome of patients with obscure gastrointestinal bleeding after capsule endoscopy: report of 100 consecutive cases. Gastroenterology 2004;126:643–53.

13. Zaman A, Katon RM. Push enteroscopy for obscure gastrointestinal bleeding yields a high incidence of proximal lesions within reach of a standard endoscope. Gastrointest Endosc 1998;47:372–6.

14. Descamps C, Schmit A, Van Gossum A. "Missed" upper gastrointestinal tract lesions may explain "occult" bleeding. Endoscopy 1999;31:452–5.

15. Lara LF, Bloomfeld RS, Pineau BC. The rate of lesions found within reach of esophagogastroduodenoscopy during push enteroscopy depends on the type of obscure gastrointestinal bleeding. Endoscopy 2005;37:745–50.

16. Fry LC, Bellutti M, Neumann H, et al. Incidence of bleeding lesions within reach of conventional upper and lower endoscopes in patients undergoing double-balloon enteroscopy for obscure gastrointestinal bleeding. Aliment Pharmacol Ther 2009;29:342–9.

17. van Turenhout ST, Jacobs MA, van Weyenberg SJ, et al. Diagnostic yield of capsule endoscopy in a tertiary hospital in patients with obscure gastrointestinal bleeding. J Gastrointestin Liver Dis 2010;19:141–5.

18. Lorenceau-Savale C, Ben-Soussan E, Ramirez S, et al. Outcome of patients with obscure gastrointestinal bleeding after negative capsule endoscopy: results of a one-year follow-up study. Gastroenterol Clin Biol 2010;34:606–11.

19. Robinson CA, Jackson C, Condon D, et al. Impact of inpatient status and gender on small-bowel capsule endoscopy findings. Gastrointest Endosc 2011;74: 1061–6.

Moving?

Make sure your subscription moves with you!

To notify us of your new address, find your **Clinics Account Number** (located on your mailing label above your name), and contact customer service at:

Email: **journalscustomerservice-usa@elsevier.com**

800-654-2452 (subscribers in the U.S. & Canada)
314-447-8871 (subscribers outside of the U.S. & Canada)

Fax number: **314-447-8029**

Elsevier Health Sciences Division
Subscription Customer Service
3251 Riverport Lane
Maryland Heights, MO 63043

*To ensure uninterrupted delivery of your subscription, please notify us at least 4 weeks in advance of move.

Printed and bound by CPI Group (UK) Ltd, Croydon, CR0 4YY

08/05/2025

01864696-0006